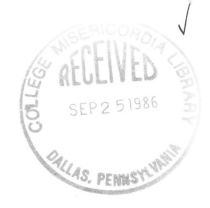

HEALTH CARE LABOR RELATIONS

A GUIDE FOR THE '80s

HEALTH CARE LABOR RELATIONS

A GUIDE FOR THE '80s

BY RENE LALIBERTY
& W. I. CHRISTOPHER
FOREWORD BY NORMAN METZGER

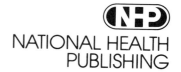

NATIONAL HEALTH
PUBLISHING

CONTENTS

PART I

HISTORY OF CHANGING EMPLOYER-EMPLOYEE RELATIONS 1

CHAPTER 1

Introduction to Labor Relations in Health
Care Facilities 5

CHAPTER 2

The Health Care Employee--An Assessment 15

CHAPTER 3

Positive Supervisory Practices to Maintain Nonunion
Status in a Health Care Facility 23

CHAPTER 4

The Substance of Labor Relations: Critical Factors 33

CHAPTER 5

Confrontation, Conflict, or Collaboration and Cooperation? . . 37

CHAPTER 6

The Governing Board: Last Step in Internal Control
for a Health Care Facility Labor Relations Program 41

PART II

MANAGEMENT AND THE UNION 51

CHAPTER 7

The Union: Friend or Foe to Management? 55

PART III

FOREWORD

Thirteen years ago I co-authored one of the earliest books on Labor Relations in the Health Care Field, *Labor-Management Relations in the Health Services Industry: Theory and Practice.* It was an attempt to introduce a much-discussed and little-understood responsibility that indeed had many negative overtones. At that time, health care unions were becoming more and more powerful, and the chroniclers of doom predicted the widespread organization of hospitals and health care facilities.

On August 25, 1974, as one of his last acts in office, President Richard M. Nixon signed the health care institutions amendments to the National Labor Relations Act. These amendments covered some 1.4 million employees who had previously been exempted from the NLRA. In the past 11 years we have seen a proliferation of National Labor Relations Board decisions, augmented by decisions of our highest courts. We have witnessed a developing sophistication on the part of health care managements towards Labor Relations.

It is within this context--the rising challenge of unions to the nonunion status of the majority of health care institutions, the strategically planned responses by management to maintain nonunion status, and the change in the perception of unions in the United States over the past several years--that the authors of this book present to us a much-needed review of where we were, where we are, and where we are going in the field of labor relations. Too few authors are willing to accept the challenge of such a review. Most are content to focus their attention on specialized, limited arenas of the problem. So we see a proliferation of books on the grievance procedure, on strikes, on maintaining nonunion status, on the law. But too few opportunities are afforded practitioners, managers, and supervisors to have under one cover a book with a Gestalt approach.

The approach taken in *Health Care Labor Relations: A Guide for the 80s* is down-to-earth. This excellent book will help health care management personnel at all levels deal with the complex and difficult roles into which they are thrust when dealing with labor relations or personnel practices. It is an excellent reference source for those who may find themselves dealing with union organizational attempts, grievance administration, and the entire collective bargaining process. The challenge to health care institutions from union organizational efforts must be addressed. This arena has not been over-studied or overpublished. It is dynamic and volatile, and it is essential that health care management understand what has happened and what to expect as a result of the inclusion of their institutions in the coverage of the National Labor Relations Act.

The authors are to be commended for looking at both sides of the coin: 1) living with unions, and 2) maintaining nonunion status. Living with unions is a complex and ever changing situation. There is a constant need to reevaluate approaches and practices, since they often become brittle in the light of the changing context of the law, its interpretation, and employee perceptions. Maintaining nonunion status is the supreme challenge of health care administrations who wish to deal directly with their employees, and who wish to address their employee needs and concerns within the institution.

This book comes at a most propitious time in labor relations in the United States. Not since the early days of the Wagner Act have unions been so challenged and so threatened. The pendulum--ubiquitous in the fortunes of administrations, as well as in the fortunes of unions--has swung, let us say, to the right. Unions are being hard tested in certification elections. Decertification elections have proliferated to a point never before witnessed. Concession bargaining has become the rule. Public opinion of unions is at its lowest in many decades. In a Gallup poll, only 26 percent of the respondents said that they had a great deal of confidence in unions. It is apparent that the combined tide of public and business opinion is running strongly against organized labor. But juxtaposed to these startling developments and the myriad of statistics showing the decline in the union movement, unions have been somewhat more successful in the health care industry and still consider it a primary and vulnerable target. Management has been quick to assert itself and has undertaken bold, well-planned and, indeed, well-received campaigns to maintain nonunion status in institutions that have not been organized and to lessen the power of unions--especially in the area of work rules and benefits--in institutions that are organized. The trend towards unionization, although stalled, has not been stopped. Union organizing has now been met with aggressive, progressive, competitive positioning by health care institutions so that they are in a better position to resist it. It is a primary responsibility of health care managers to understand how they play a role in this arena.

Health Care Labor Relations: A Guide for the 80s answers the need for all levels of health care managers who wish to be better equipped in this area. As the authors point out, it was not easy for health care administrators to accept the new responsibilities imposed by the National Labor Relations Act. But accept they must. Knowledge is a powerful weapon, and knowledge is what is distributed in this book.

Norman Metzger
Edmond A. Guggenheim Professor
Department of Health Care Management
Mount Sinai School of Medicine

Vice-President for Labor Relations
The Mount Sinai Medical Center
New York, NY

PREFACE

After approximately 15 years (1968-1983) of runaway inflation, the United States health care industry was forced to cut costs.

In April 1983, President Ronald Reagan signed into law the Social Security Amendments of 1983, Public Law 98-21. In addition to overhauling the Social Security Program, the law completely restructured the Medicare system for reimbursing inpatient acute care services through the creation of a prospective payment system (PPS). PPS is based on the concept of paying hospitals a fixed price (rate-per-discharge) for 468 different categories of illness, called diagnosis related groups (DRGs). Because of the cost containment potential the new reimbursement concept embodied, strong support came forward from other sectors of the economy. As a result, institutions began facing increased pressure from private payers, including commercial insurance companies, and from private industry, to extend the DRG concept to nonfederal patients.

As a result of the federal PPS and, in many states, mandated cost control legislation advocating shorter patient stays and fewer admissions, hospitals today are facing problems of staff reductions, layoffs, and possible closure due to reductions in volume and revenue.

To enhance their positions and minimize financial risks, hospitals are strengthening internal management control systems, employing new capital acquisition strategies, strengthening and improving medical staff relationships, improving the quality and competency of their governing boards, and either merging with other local hospitals or becoming part of multihospital systems. In addition, to preclude financial failure, hospitals are developing strategic planning processes. The word "marketing" in hospitals today is as common as the words "hospital bed;" indeed, in the final analysis marketing has helped replace sources of revenue previously received from occupied hospital beds.

In the broadening of efforts to market health care differently, many American health care workers now find themselves out of the traditional acute care hospital setting and into new work environments, such as:

- Self-care teaching programs

- Home care services

- Hospice

- Outpatient surgery

- Health maintenance organizations (HMO)

- Preferred provider organizations (PPO)

- Adult day care services

- Sexual dysfunction treatment centers

- Alcohol/drug detoxification programs

- Home dialysis

- Psychiatric programs and counseling services

- Congregate housing programs

- Long-term care programs

- Skilled nursing facilities

- Emergi-centers

- Rehabilitation programs

- Wellness programs

- Mobile health services for older persons

- Entrepreneurial ventures

- Family respite centers

- Home emergency programs

- Stress and mental health centers

- Birthing centers

The issues for the American health care system, are many, and they are complex. They are the same from coast to coast, in rural and urban, small and large health care institutions[1]. The issues are:

- Mandated cost controls from the federal and/or state governments

- Competition for limited amounts of health care dollars

- Quality of service(s)

- Competency and productivity of staff

- Job security in view of reductions in force and layoffs

- Labor force changes and their affect on unionization and/or employee relations

- Organizational restructuring into a corporate mold, multi-systems or mergers

- Staffing patterns as they relate to professional versus technical, part-time versus full-time, or the advantages and disadvantages of contract services

- Continued demand from the public for top quality hospital services at reduced prices.

The onus is clearly on health care executives to guide the industry through the difficult years ahead. As the government and the public continue to demand reductions in the cost of health care services, health care executives will increasingly find themselves facing unique human resource problems. To all of its economic and social complexities the American health care industry is now adding reductions in force, layoffs, changes in organizational structure, and the need to find new markets for its services. These new dimensions will in some institutions cause employees to take more of an interest in unionization or other job actions. Health care executives have an opportunity at this point to design an effective and long-lasting human resource strategic planning process for their institutions. However, in order for their efforts to be both credible and fruitful, they will need to place more of an emphasis on people.

In a capitalist society it is not surprising that there is a major concentration on money. Yet in a democratic society it is somewhat surprising that there is not an equal emphasis and importance on people. Unfortunately, sometimes money speaks. And too often we do not focus on the human element.

It would be a very trite statement to say that quality patient care lies in the people who provide it. All the other factors with which management must deal to run a modern health care facility are available equally. Each can seek the newest equipment, buy the same supply items, use the same techniques and systems. The difference in what one health care facility does and what another health care facility does not do is not in the equipment, the machines, or the item; it is in the people who have been recruited, developed, retained, and motivated to achieve appropriate results.

There are good health care facilities and there are poor health care facilities. The difference eventually comes down to people, what they do, and how they are managed. Therefore, it is important that one of management's priorities be human resources.

People are complex beings. Personnel placement per se, as one part of a comprehensive human resource program, will always be the same old square peg and square hole task. It won't change. It will still entail bringing together the right worker and the right job. However, a comprehensive human resource program adds other ingredients--a point that has been long-ignored. The other ingredients involve the atmosphere in which you place the job and the worker: the physical setting, the economic setting, the social setting, the managerial setting, and the psychological setting. If these environments are positive, people will mature, be encouraged, and feel motivated to do what management wants done. And that is when a human resource program excels.

Managers of health care facilities, or major departments of health care facilities, find themselves today dependent on a group that must be moved in a new direction to do what they want done in order for the facility to survive. Too often managers react to employees instead of employees reacting to management. There are many philosophies and approaches to the overall concept of management and of human resource management. But regardless of the approach taken in human resource management, all the elements need to be interrelated and interdependent. It is not possible to take a few of the pieces, apply them, and await total results. If an electronics engineer decided to build a stereo set and ordered a do-it-yourself kit, he wouldn't sit there and say, "I think I'll leave out this tube and that transistor," and expect to get high fidelity sound reproduction. Yet many chief executive officers do sit back in a health care facility and say, "I don't think we'll take the time to do a morale survey." "I don't think it's important that we set up good personnel policies and practices." "Who cares if the employees unionize?" "Perhaps we shouldn't evaluate personnel." These same executives then expect overall long-range full results from their human resource department.

In a sense, the whole is greater than the sum of its parts. This is an old psychological phenomenon, but it applies fully to the field of human resource management. All the parts will create a human resource program. All the parts will create better results in achieving the goals of the institution.

The purpose of this book is to provide health care executives and governing board members with the most relevant, timely, and comprehensive information available on labor relations and personnel administration matters. A distinguishing feature of the book is that special attention is directed to the managerial environment as it relates to improved or disrupted labor relations. A review of the consequences of failure of management to be receptive and responsive to the clues of deteriorating morale and negative employee relations will stimulate in the reader greater interest in the positive aspects of a voluntary labor relations program without the collective bargaining process.

Unlike novels, textbooks are rarely read from cover to cover. Readers use professional and technical literature for research, education, or to obtain information about specific subjects. Authors of professional and technical literature, in their anxiety to create successful books, frequently try to incorporate into their work novel theories or concepts that will attract and hold the attention of the reader. In preparing the material for this book, our main objective was to consolidate only practical and useful information about labor relations and personnel administration as they relate to the health care industry.

We hope our contribution will be considered a consultant adjunct for chief executive officers, governing boards, vice-presidents, directors of human resource management, directors of education and training, various department directors, assistant directors in clinical staff and support areas, and as text for educational programs. The contents of this book are applicable to both union and nonunion facilities, and the material is relevant for non-profit or governmental entities.[2]

This book is not another text on dealing with organized labor, nor does it go deeply into the specifics of labor relations law. It is instead a more comprehensive examination based on practical experiences of the larger issue of internal labor relations in health care facilities. It is not expected to solve all problems nor is it intended to serve as a substitute for experienced and competent labor relations counsel in any dealings with employees, unions, or union activity. It will, however, point out specific concerns in dealing with labor and employee relations issues with or without union involvement.

For those already involved with organized labor groups and collective bargaining agreements, focus is directed to some of the critical issues that should receive management's attention to retain control appropriate to the responsibilities assumed.

The book also has a case study of a four-week total union campaign leading to a National Labor Relations Board representation election. The purpose of this case study is to give the reader a deeper insight to critical issues that often swing the employee's attention and his/her vote.

It is hoped that the content of this text will well serve the interests of health care management at all levels in their quest for interdependent cooperation to provide the essential aspects of quality care to the patients, who often become the innocent victims of failing labor relations within health care facilities.

Rene Laliberty
Waterville, Maine

W. I. Christopher
Gulf Shores, Alabama

---

1. For ease of presentation, we will employ the terms "health care institution," "facility," and "entity;" in most instances the material is equally applicable to various forms of health care delivery institutions (e.g., hospitals, nursing homes, clinics, health maintenance organizations, neighborhood health centers, etc.)

2. Health care facilities are of three types, for-profit institutions/privately owned; nonprofit organizations; and governmental. The private, for-profit health care facilities operate like any business enterprise. A for-profit organization's prime concern is to operate at a profit, which in essence represents return on investment for investors. A nonprofit health care facility has no investors and has as its primary concern the provision of service to the patient, i.e., responsibility to the society in which it functions. However, it must remain solvent in order to provide that service. Profits generated in a nonprofit institution are kept within the facility as operating capital. Governmental institutions are operated under the jurisdiction of either the federal government or a state government.

ACKNOWLEDGMENTS

Our special thanks to Donna Gordon and to Joan MacKenzie from the Personnel Department of the Mid-Maine Medical Center, who carefully assimilated our manuscript and really kept us on schedule to meet the publisher's deadline requirements.

We are deeply indebted to Joseph J. Bean, Jr., Senior Associate, John Christie Associates, Augusta, Maine, for permitting us to use some of the material from a book he co-authored (*Understanding Hospital Labor Relations*--Reading, MA: Addison-Wesley, 1977). Thank you, Joe.

We would also like to acknowledge the assistance and contribution of those who took part in the preparation of this book.

V. Brandon Melton
Society Director
American Society for
Hospital Personnel
Administration
American Hospital Association
Chicago, IL

Norman Metzger
Vice President - Labor
Relations
Mt. Sinai Medical Center
New York, NY

Judy Minkove
Developmental Editor
Rynd Communications
Owings Mills, MD

Jacqueline Karkos
Vice President
Rynd Communications
Owings Mills, MD

Barbara Bloom Kreml
Director
Dept. of Human Resources
American Hospital Assoc.
Chicago, IL

Elanore Lampner
Acquisitions Editor
Rynd Communications
Owings Mills, MD

Chapter 8 "Basic Components of the Union Election Process: Bargaining Units and Decertification" was edited and critiqued by Duane R. Batista from the law firm of Nutter, McClennen, & Fish, Boston, Massachusetts.

Chapter 10, "The Collective Bargaining Process" was edited and critiqued by Peter Jacobs from the law firm of Pierce, Atwood, Scribner, Allen, Smith & Lancaster, Portland, Maine.

Special thanks to John Sheridan Associates, Inc. and its subsidiary Human Resource Services, Inc., Carmel, California, for allowing us to use their Employee Attitude Survey entitled "Viewpoint."

We are indebted to both Duane Batista and Peter Jacobs for helping us with Chapters 8 and 10.

ABOUT THE AUTHORS

W. I. Christopher is the founder and principal of Management Enterprises, St. Louis, Missouri and Gulf Shores, Alabama, a firm of consultants for hospitals, nursing homes, service institutions, and businesses, with major emphasis in the fields of management, supervision, personnel, and public relations. Mr. Christopher developed many projects and services in management, supervision, personnel, and public relations, including a unique method of management improvement training for supervisors utilizing short-interval taped presentations in a group therapy and group dynamics setting. He is author of over 100 articles, leaflets, manuals, and texts.

Rene Laliberty is Vice President for Personnel and Employee Relations, Mid-Maine Medical Center, Waterville, Maine. He is co-author of three books dealing with labor relations, hospital management, and health care productivity. He has twice won the annual award for literature given by the American Society for Healthcare Human Resources Administration. He is a frequent speaker and writer. Most noteworthy are recent speaking and writing engagements in Australia as the United States representative at several Australian Hospital Association meetings. Mr. Laliberty is a board member of the National Commission for Health Certifying Agencies. He is also the immediate past President of the American Society for Healthcare Human Resources Administration, and is the 1986 recipient of their Distinguished Achievement Award. He has been actively working with the Voluntary Hospitals of America, Inc. in creating a national Corporate Human Resource function for the Voluntary Hospitals of America.

PART I

HISTORY OF CHANGING EMPLOYER-EMPLOYEE RELATIONS

INTRODUCTION

HISTORY OF CHANGING EMPLOYER-EMPLOYEE RELATIONS

This first section of the book gives an overview of why health care facilities are atypical organizations. It presents a look at how and why a "people" industry has traditionally ignored employee relations. The chapters in Part One will introduce the reader to labor relations in health care facilities, the changes in traditional health care employee roles, the corporate changes taking place in the American health care system, and the struggle to move from a management style created a generation ago to a more modern style needed for the future.

Part One also depicts the effects the Medicare Prospective Payment System, Diagnosis Related Groups (DRGs) have had on health care facilities and unions. It concludes with a chapter on the governing board, the last step in internal control for a health care facility labor relations program.

CHAPTER 1

Introduction to Labor Relations in Health Care Facilities

Health care facilities are not typical corporations, particularly in the area of labor relations. As Ray Brown explains:

> The hospital was originally conceived as an agency dedicated to doing good rather than well. It was little more than a home away from home for the sick poor. The physicians did not need the hospital in the beginning and the hospital didn't need management. Money was almost the sole problem of the early hospital and it was not a serious one. The persons who put up the needed sums of money thereby solved the major problem. These persons were the trustees, and they sat alone in the governance saddle because they were responsible for the saddle-bags.[1]

Over the years, the American health care delivery system has changed more dramatically than any other kind of corporation. The health care field has transformed itself from a small philanthropic endeavor of the 1800s to a megacorporate system. The changes generated from within the health care field have been nothing less than spectacular.

During this same period of time, health care facilities, both acute and long-term care, have had to react to and change with social changes much more dramatically than has private industry. These changes in the scope and nature of the services provided are the results of the influences and pressures mandated by the community, industrial employers, and the state and federal governments.

The primary purpose of the more than 7,000 hospitals and 18,000 nursing homes in the United States is to meet the major health and long-term care needs of the population. Their major functions include caring for the sick and the elderly, promoting public and professional education, conducting medical research, and practicing preventive medicine.

Rapid medical and technological advances have greatly upgraded medical care. The average stay in an acute care facility per illness has been reduced from 58 days in the 1870s (when charges for hospital care were actually computed by the week) to approximately 7 days at present. The technology now available has made diagnosis and treatment more rapid than was thought possible a hundred years ago.

It is estimated by Beverly Enterprises of Pasadena, California, the nation's largest nursing home chain, that an additional 169,000 nursing home beds will be needed by 1990 to keep pace with the rapidly growing number of people over 65.

Currently, approximately 5.6 percent of persons age 65 and older live in nursing homes. The long-term care industry is rapidly developing alternative systems of care--such as congregate living and home health care to meet the growing and diverse needs of our elderly population.

To achieve these breakthroughs, health care facilities have been forced to grow in size, complexity, and, of course, expense. As a result, today's health care complexes are acknowledged as big businesses. As the systems grew, so did public skepticism. Health care costs and related stories of inadequate care led many to see health care facilities as institutions of private rather than public interest. As health care facilities continue to assume more responsibility for overall public health, they will become an even greater part of the public plan. The public will want to have a greater say in their development and operation. Thus, hospitals and nursing homes will not be able to achieve their objectives except as an integral part of the total effort directed toward improvement of the health and welfare of the communities they serve. To this end, hospitals and long-term care facilities have a vital role to play which can be accomplished only by an efficiently run facility staffed by skilled, dedicated, and reliable employees.

Many skills, all of which are important, are necessary in the operation of a medical or long-term care facility. Supervisors, who are the liaison between the facility and the community, patient and staff, employee and management, are especially vital members of the health care team. Jonathon Rakich thus aptly describes the community general hospital as "an organization that mobilizes the skills and efforts of a number of widely divergent groups of professional, semiprofessional, and nonprofessional personnel to provide a highly personalized service to individual patients. Like other large-scale organizations, it is established and designed to pursue certain objectives through collaborative activity."[2] Therefore, the supervisor's role is both difficult and crucial in the operation of a medical facility.

Professor Basil S. Georgopoulos has concluded that since health care is a "people industry," one cannot equate labor relations matters in health care with labor relations functions in industry. Hospital work, for example, is carried out by numerous cooperating people where backgrounds, education, training, skills, and functions are as diverse and heterogenous as the most complex organizations on record.[3]

While employees in all cases deserve and seek recognition of their bargaining rights vis-a-vis management, the goals of the institutions they work for are often vastly different. Industrial management aims principally at maximization of profit; health care management aims principally at maximization of meeting community health care needs, some for profit and some not for profit. Unlike many organizations, health care facilities are able to make the role they perform in the community psychologically meaningful to their employees. And most health care employees give unselfishly of their energies to perform the tasks assigned to them. Most staff members, both professional and nonprofessional, consider their work very important and find working in a health care facility deeply satisfying. They do not, however, always recognize the unique difference from other corporate structures in terms of nonprofit or profit ownership.

"It is also interesting and important to note that unlike industrial and other large-scale organizations, [health care facilities] rely very heavily on the integrity, skills, motivations, and behaviors of its members for the attainment of its objectives. The flow of work in a hospital is too variable and too irregular to permit mechanical standardization."[3] Because the work cannot be planned in advance with the automatic precision of an assembly line, the facility must depend on its employees to make the day-to-day adjustments that the work situation may demand. This adjustment factor may go from a 50 percent census period of relative inactivity to a spontaneous 100 percent census period of spasmodic action. All of these factors necessitate heavy reliance on the employees to coordinate their activities on a voluntary, informal, and expedient basis.

"Fundamentally, then, [health care facilities] are human systems rather than machine-like systems. Even though they may possess elaborate and impressive looking equipment or a great variety of physical and material facilities, they have no real integrated mechanical system for the handling and processing of their work."[3] They must rely heavily on the human element for the accomplishment of their primary reason for existence: patient care, people caring for people. "However, as paradoxical as it may seem, [health care facilities] are also highly formal, quasi-bureaucratic organization which, like all task-oriented organizations, relies a great deal upon formal written rules and regulations and formal authority for controlling much of the behavior and work relationships of its members. This emphasis on formal procedures and on directives rather than 'democratic' controls, along with a number of other factors, gives [health care facilities] their much talked about 'authoritarian' character. Lines of authority and responsibility must be clearly drawn, and basic acceptance of authority must be assured. When human life is at stake, there is little tolerance for error or negligence."[3] If errors and negligence can be prevented by adherence to strict formal rules and dictatorial discipline, such rules are important to have and cannot very well be questioned. (We're not talking now about blind obedience-- because the hospital increasingly relies on the expertise, judgment, and ethics of professionals who, while abhorring regimentation, are capable of a great deal of self-discipline.)

"[Health care facilities] are expected to be able to provide adequate care to their patients at all times with the snap of precision of a machine and with a minimum of error. Even though they have an error-prone human system to rely upon, they are expected to perform well continuously and to produce with machine-like response toward the patient regardless of such things as turnover, absenteeism, feelings of hostility among their personnel, or labor relations problems that they may be experiencing."[3]

Another of the distinctive labor relations complexities in a health care facility is the absence of a single line of authority. Essentially authority is shared by a governing board, the director of personnel, the director of operations, the director of finance, the director of nursing, the doctors, and the chief executive officer--these are the major centers of influence in a health care institution.

The governing board delegates the day-to-day management to the chief executive officer. In turn, the chief executive officer delegates authority to the heads of the various departments. On the formal organizational chart, the medical staff, its officers, and the members are not shown as having any direct-line responsibility; they are outside the lay-administration line of authority. "Yet, it is well known that doctors exercise substantial influence throughout the facility at nearly all levels. They enjoy very high autonomy in their work and have a good deal of professional authority over employees in the institution. Although the governing board is the ultimate source of authority, the Board actually has very limited de facto authority over the medical staff. This is partly because the doctors are not employees of the hospital (they are 'guests' who are granted practice privileges), and partly because they enjoy high status and great prestige. The doctors have almost supreme authority in professional-medical matters and are subject to very little lay-organizational authority."[3]

In general, the many lines of authority require a very delicate balance of power in a health care facility,[3] a balance of power that is rather precarious from a labor relations point of view. As Metzger and Pointer note:

> The development of employee organization in health care facilities dates from 1919, although sustained activity was not initiated until the late 1930s. Up until 1972 union activity was mostly confined to geographically isolated areas of the country, primarily the East and West coasts, and certain portions of the Midwest. Recognition has appeared to be the primary obstacle to collective activity in hospitals. The success of Local 1199 in organizing in New York City hospitals during the 1960s established a solid foundation on which to expand.[4]

In 1974, Congress enacted Public Law No. 93-360 amending the National Labor Relations Act (NLRA) and expanding jurisdiction of the National Labor Relations Board (NLRB) to cover for the first time employees of nonprofit hospitals. Prior to 1974, the NLRA expressly excluded from the definition of "employer" any corporation or association operating a hospital, if no part of the net earnings inured to the benefit of any private shareholder or individual. The 1974 amendment deleted this exclusion, thus bringing nonprofit hospitals within the definition of "employer" and within the coverage of NLRA.

Because Congress was aware of the importance of preventing disruption of patient care while allowing hospital employees the protections of the NLRA, the 1974 amendments also added the special limitations and protections that apply to "health care institutions." The NLRA as amended defined a health care institution as including any hospital, convalescent hospital, health maintenance organization, health clinic, nursing home, extended care facility, or other institution devoted to the care of the sick, infirm, or aged persons.

Employers within the definition of "health care institution" were afforded special protections under the NLRA to minimize the number of strikes occurring in health care facilities and to allow employers, in the event of a dispute, sufficient notice to make arrangements for the care of patients. For example, in approving bargaining units of health care employees, the NLRB is subject to a congressional mandate to prevent proliferation of bargaining units. Health care institutions are also entitled to a special 10-day written notice of a strike or other concerted activity under section 8(g) of the NLRA. Health care institutions and unions are also subject to special notice requirements under section 8(d) concerning termination or modification of a collective bargaining agreement. Where bargaining is for an initial agreement, the union must give notice of a dispute before it can give a 10-day strike notice. Mandatory mediation between a health care institution and a labor organization may be required at the request of the Federal Mediation and Conciliation Service (FMCS).

Some of the facilities included within the statutory definition of "health care institution" were already subject to the NLRB jurisdiction prior to 1974, as the exclusion deleted in 1974 applied only to nonprofit hospitals. The NLRB had elected in some cases not to exercise its full statutory authority over other nonprofit health care and human service providers. Since 1974, the Board has expanded its exercise of jurisdiction over all health care institutions and other human service providers.

With the coverage of nonprofit health care facilities under the 1974 amendments to NLRA, management in the health industry was required to deal collectively with its employees. Many were required to operate under the new law with no prior experience, and a major concern developed that collective bargaining would deprive management of its flexibility in dealing with employees. The 1974 amendments to the NLRA opened for the unions an opportunity to capitalize on employee dissatisfaction and forced management to reexamine its employee relations policies.

Two labor relations writers have concluded:

> There is no greater threat facing the health care industry today than the spread of the union epidemic. According to the National Labor Relations Board unions won only forty-eight percent of the total board-conducted elections in 1975. This, the board reports, is the lowest percentage of union victories in the board's forty-year history. The health care industry, however, did not fare so well. Between August, 1974 and the end of April 1975, the union success in the health care industry elections was sixty-two percent. Strikes, slowdowns, and

other work stoppages threatened the very core of health care in such states as New York, Hawaii, California, and Texas.[5]

Public opinion toward the collective rights of health care employees has been reconsidered. Collective organizational rights of fire fighters, police officers, schoolteachers, professional athletes, and interns have caused a rethinking of the rights of institutional employees to become unionized.

By the inclusion of health care facilities in the 1974 NLRA amendments, approximately 4,000 hospitals and 18,000 nursing homes were brought under the jurisdiction of the National Labor Relations Board. It is no wonder that the management in these hospitals and nursing homes were alarmed. Not only did they not know what the effects of the 1974 NLRA amendments relative to unionization would be, but in most cases they did not entirely know what they could or could not do to either prevent or soften unionization attempts in their institutions.

For the most part, it was not easy for health care administrators to accept the new responsibilities imposed by the NLRA. More storm clouds were forming that would further test the tenacity of the American health care system.

During the 1970s and early 1980s, the nation's hospital bill was rising at annual rates as high as 19 percent. One major engine driving this seemingly unstoppable surge was Medicare, the federal health insurance program for the elderly that was created in 1965 and covered approximately 40 percent of all hospital admissions.

Between 1971 and 1982 Medicare costs zoomed from $7.5 billion to $50 billion under an open-ended payment system, pushing up costs for all health care consumers in the process. Some strong medicine was prescribed by Congress in the form of Diagnosis Related Groups (DRGs), which became a component of the Prospective Payment System (PPS). Congress set up 468 illness categories, each with a predetermined payment. Hospitals that treated a Medicare patient for less than standard payment could keep the difference as a profit. Those who spent more would have to absorb the difference.

On October 1, 1983, Medicare began implementing its prospective payment system (PPS) for acute hospital inpatient services. That shift from a cost-based to a fixed-price system caused major financial and labor relations problems for some hospitals. Although PPS applied only to Medicare, it was a revolutionary change with far-reaching labor implications. For the first time, the health care industry in the United States would have to assume financial risk in exchange for its payments under the Medicare program.

While Medicare was the first insurer to implement that concept on a national basis, many states began experimenting or developed systems designed to achieve the same objectives. Other insurers, under pressure from employers and the public, also began sending messages to health care providers that they no longer could support ever-increasing health care insurance premiums. It thus became clear to health care providers that if they wished to remain financially viable, they would have to develop tools to manage resource consumption on a per-case basis.

Previously, the basis for payment for most third-party payors was the hospital's reasonable cost or billed charges. In that kind of a financial environment, the major role of the health care facility was to maximize revenues to support the medical and operational decisions made by the governing boards, administration, and the medical staff.

Because salary dollars in the health care industry represent a major portion of the operating budget, a reexamination of all aspects of staffing and labor complements became mandatory. Also, business, stung by high health insurance premiums, started changing health insurance coverages so that employees would have an incentive to use inpatient hospital services less. As inpatient utilization rates in hospitals began to fall, an action, foreign to most hospitals, began to happen: reduction in force, also known as layoffs.

It is generally conceded that working conditions and wages in health care facilities have never really kept pace with those in other industries. Health care management for many years was successful in advocating that the health care industry was serving humanity, and for many institutions that was enough to explain away any wage and benefit disparities. The rationale worked very well for the health care industry, especially when coupled with the appeal that the health care facility gave its employees unparalleled job security.

Just as the 1974 amendments to the NLRA caused a labor relations shock wave for hospital administrators, prospective payment systems and other mandated state health care cost controls caused a similar shock wave in 1983 for health care employees in that they eroded, for the first time, the employees' job security.

Service Employees International Union (SEIU), representing 210,000 hospital workers in the United States, saw in 1983 for the first time layoffs of its hospital members in Michigan, Ohio, and the Pacific Northwest. State and metropolitan hospital associations began reporting lack-of-work separations in January 1983. The American Hospital Association data began to indicate that admissions had declined 3.4 percent in the first quarter of 1983 compared to the first quarter of 1982. The layoff trend became systemwide throughout the country as hospitals streamlined their staffs to fit a decreased work load.

Nursing homes are now serving sicker patients because of the growing number of frail elderly. Medicare's prospective payment system also encourages hospitals to discharge recovering patients to the less-costly nursing home environment. As a result, the long-term care industry cannot keep pace with the demand for nursing home beds. This demand necessitates, in most cases, that nursing homes enforce limitations and reserve available beds for the sickest patients. Although the demand for nursing home beds and special care needs results in increased revenues for nursing homes, it will present labor problems for the long-term care facilities.

During the next 10 years, job security for hospital health care employees will be the main issue in labor relations. Union organizing will focus on employee perception of whether or not the hospital in question can reduce labor complements fairly. If management and labor cannot negotiate the job security concern, then job security will become a major strike issue in health care facilities.

During the next five years, the shortage of nursing home beds and the transfer of sicker patients to long-term care facilities will create for that segment of the American health care system requests for additional professional staff and improvements in the wage and benefits systems. In this era of attempts to eliminate discrimination in our society, it is not unrealistic to expect that health care workers will demand equal rights and attack any perceived injustices related to their employment.

The plight of health care employees in a complex organizational structured work environment, coupled with their rights under the NLRA plus the economic squeeze that the American health care system will be experiencing for the next decade, will present for the American health care system an increase in labor relation activities. That prospect could jeopardize the delivery of care for the American public.

From the point of view of meeting the responsibility of an effective operation of a health care facility in today's and tomorrow's health care environment, there are sound reasons for management to pursue and maintain an effective and direct relationship with employees.

ENDNOTES

1. Ray E. Brown. *Hospital Organization and Management.* 1972. The Catholic Hospital Association.

2. Jonathan S. Rakich. *Hospital Organization and Management.* 1972. The Catholic Hospital Association.

3. Basil S. Georgopoulos, Ph.D. (Research Scientist, Program Director, and Professor of Psychology at the University of Michigan) and Floyd C. Mann, Ph.D. (Environmental Council, University of Colorado) completed an extensive analysis of "The Hospital as an Organization." New York: Macmillan Company, July, 1962.

4. Norman Metzger, and Dennis D. Pointer. *Labor Management Relations in the Health Care Services Industry.* Source Book Series, Vol. 4, New York: Science & Health Publication, 1972.

5. Warren H. Chaney, and Thomas R. Beech, *The Union Epidemic*. Rockville, MD: Aspen Publication, 1976.

CHAPTER 2

The Health Care Employee — An Assessment

A MEASURE OF PROGRESS

The history of the American labor movement offers a yardstick by which one can measure the living standard and status of the American worker. Today, American workers have various forms of protection as individuals and employees, but there was a time in our history when the American worker was debased and unprotected in socioeconomic and employment matters. Industrialists of the past generally looked upon labor as a commodity or as a resource to be mined of its vitality and then discarded. Unfortunately, the health care industry (medical facilities and nursing homes) cannot be excluded from that analysis.

But the lot of the American health care worker, like that of workers in industry, has come a long way in the last 30 years. The people who care for other people--nurses, technologists, nurse aides, dietitians, social workers, food service personnel, and housekeeping staffs--now also care for themselves and are not reluctant to talk about their concerns. From the point of view of health care workers, there is not a trace of lament for the "good old days" of frustrating working conditions, low wages, and professional paradoxes.

However, neither is the present utopian. There are still areas that need improvement, such as home health agencies, long-term care facilities, health maintenance organizations (HMOs), community clinics, and regional health agencies. The wages paid to employees in these segments of the health care industry are not totally on par with the wages paid in the acute care hospital settings. Other concerns that need to be addressed are: recognition commensurate with contribution to the health care system, continuing education programs, supervisory indifference, equitable range of benefits, and in some areas, job security. For these segments of the health care industry the possibility of increased unionization attempts is a very real possibility, unless management starts bridging the inequity gaps.

An in-depth analysis of the health care workers' past reveals not only prime employee concerns related to wages, benefits, continuing education, and working conditions, but also concerns about job safety and quality of supervision. Health care employees have not always been treated equitably by supervisors or upper management. In most cases, employees were not intentionally exploited by management, but neither did management always initiate programs to meet their needs. Employees often became frustrated in their attempts to be heard.

For many years, while the cost of living soared, health care employees' wages left them behind the major portion of the American workforce.[1] Yet they

15

were always asked to serve society without complaint. Through the years, while rising costs of industrial goods had been accepted (though less than enthusiastically), the rising costs of health care met with public consternation. Health care workers frequently were forced to accept public criticism for health care costs and policy matters over which they had little or no control.

The public still feels that health care facilities are unique and, therefore, people employed in health care institutions should be treated differently from workers from other service or manufacturing industries. So, observes Dennis Kobs, "No unanimity of opinion exists, but in general hospital administrators and hospital trustees are rather conservative and try to avoid any radical change from the past."[2]

The arrival of a union is often seen as the entrance of a "knight in shining armor." In its organizing efforts, the union does more than present the workers with channels for releasing frustrations. It also promises to increase their economic well-being and offers them a vehicle for expressing their views to the public and upper management. To the employees, the union becomes a means of obtaining a voice in their destiny.

The union's record in negotiating wages and fringe benefits is frequently a key selling point in organizing attempts. The union's professed understanding of the employees' problems gives the employees a feeling of support in the sharing of a common cause with others.

When "labor," "labor relations," or "personnel relations" is mentioned to some managers, it is not unusual for them to react defensively. "This is my department; these are my people," they say. Health care supervisors call this concern an "interest in my people." Skilled labor organizers call it "paternalism." Paternalism in health care has worked well as a labor relations panacea for many years. In our opinion, however, the paternalistic approach to resolving labor matters will not work with today's typically strong confident health care workers. America's health care employees are among its most educated and technically competent people, and they should not be treated like children.

Many health care supervisors still have "tunnel vision" in recognizing their objectives. While service to patients is a primary objective, it cannot be the only objective. Health care supervisors have for a long time ignored their employees. The health care industry has allowed itself the luxury of apathy for too long a time. It has allowed employee needs to go unfulfilled and has tolerated poor departmental supervision and "henpecking"--all under the guise that public service is being performed and that supervision is secondary.

HUMAN RESOURCE MANAGEMENT TRENDS

Progress has been made in the acceptance of sound human resource programs in many health care facilities. There has been steady growth of new personnel programs--sometimes voluntarily, sometimes after a sharp jab or nudge from the employees, sometimes by the facilities after the union has whistled at them. Whatever the impetus, progress has occurred and further progress will be made as health care supervisors and upper management achieve a degree of maturity in the labor relations arena.

It has been recognized in personnel management that what an employee believes to be true is frequently much more important than what may actually be true, and that one needs to react quickly to the employees' thoughts in order to avoid a labor relations incident. If only one person in a department thinks something is true, however remote that thought may be from the actual truth, that individual can cause an effective system or institution to be mired in a sea of labor relations conflicts. The era of management in the health care industry when it was more convenient to leave controversial issues alone has passed. The new concentration is on resolving the differences quickly to preclude labor relations difficulties.

Until recent years, little attention was given to employee attitudes, behavior, management techniques, or employee participation in resolving differences. Today, there are many reasons and many pressures for an effective human resource management system in health care facilities. Employees exercise a profound influence on the institution by their conduct and attitude on the job. Employee effectiveness, as reflected in the amount and quality of work, is greatly dependent on or related to employee attitudes toward those involved in the management or operation of the institution.

Health care facilities are undergoing changes of both a corporate and functional nature. Increasingly, they are becoming more complex to operate. This change is creating important problems, not the least of which is the establishment of an effective communication system between management and employees. As leaders in labor relations, we are struggling to move from a management style created a generation ago to a modern style needed for the future, and we really don't know how to begin or how to get our people involved in the new system.

Health care management can no longer be administratively isolated. It must now be interrelated with human resource management programs to such a degree that it becomes a major program in the facility. The health care industry today is concerned about its current managerial effectiveness, and rightly so. Managers are beginning to realize that they may not be totally in command of things in the years ahead. Management's voice grows weaker as one looks from the past to the impact of the 1974 NLRA amendments on the health care industry, and beyond to future changes in the overall economic structure of the American health care system.

Workers and their work are vital managerial factors in today's and tomorrow's health care system: lose control of them, and you've lost some control of your management system. Control will remain in the hands of those who have the vision to exercise new human resource programs.

Maintaining control, however, is not simple. Today's health care workers hold a different view of the institution as a place of employment from their counterparts of two decades ago. Employees know and monitor their rights. Employees know what management can and cannot do relative to their employment status. They know that laws set forth both what must be done and what must no longer be done with regard to workers, laws that a few short years ago either did not exist or were not applicable to the health care industry. For instance, we now have laws that protect the rights of employees in the following areas:

- Wages

- Benefits

- Civil rights

- Occupational safety and health matters

- Work injury compensation

- Unemployment compensation

- Equal opportunity employment matters

- The right to organize

- Coverage under the Fair Labor Standards Act.

While today's workers are still interested in bettering their living standards and job security, they also want a piece of the action. They are no longer willing to adapt themselves to the demands of machines or to management's unilateral decisions concerning their work and professions. In short, today's workers want to manage parts of their jobs. Participatory management relationships between workers and managers in the health care field are bound to intensify . . . all the ingredients are there.

HUMAN RESOURCES IN A CHANGING ENVIRONMENT

The economic environment, corporate structures, and marketing needs of the American health care system have been changing with accelerating speed. But the developments have generally not included mechanisms for letting management know how employees feel about the changing scene. As a result, developments in the human resource sphere lag behind; and as long as that is the case, there will be fertile ground for increased unionization. Whatever we do to control costs and change the system, we must not do it at the expense of the human resource factors.

Twenty years ago, labor relations, employee relations, and personnel administration functions rarely existed in the American health care system--and where they did, they were typically run by people with some administrative talent who performed routine tasks such as interviewing and recruiting. Today, human resource management functions need highly skilled professionals capable of guiding management in an increasingly inhibiting and complex legal environment. As mentioned in the previous chapter, the unparalleled job security that health care employees have enjoyed for three decades is eroding due to the influence of DRGs, increased competition for the available health care dollar, and other mandated cost control legislation. These factors are causing a decline in inpatient volumes in the health industry and contributing to an overall economic downturn. Job security is a new concern for health care employees whether unionized or not. For the unionized, it could be a major strike issue. For the health care facilities that are nonunion, employees most likely will push for some form of job guarantee or seek to become unionized in order to achieve or enhance their job security.

As an example, for nearly a century, employers in almost every state have had the right to discharge so-called "at-will employees." Their discharge can be either with or without cause.[3] This common-law doctrine of employment was first used in a Pennsylvania court in 1891. It covers employees who are either not covered by a collective bargaining contract, not employed under a written employment contract, or not covered by any socioeconomic protective legislation, that is, laws that prohibit termination based on race, sex, age, religion, or similar criteria. Those not protected by any of the above can be discharged for any or no reason, hence the title "at-will." The vast majority of American health care workers are "at-will" employees. Less than 25 percent of the health care industry work force is under union contracts; therefore, few have written employment contracts. Health care workers without union contracts will be more apt to look for some kind of protection, and they may look to the courts for broader protection against termination for economic reasons, which would mean an erosion of the long-standing employment-at-will doctrine.

Employees view job security as one of the principal benefits of unionization. If the courts eventually do guarantee job security, then the changes in the "at-will" doctrine could become an effective management tool to counter union organizing efforts if used properly. Successful court cases challenging employers' right to terminate "at-will" employees for any or no reason have been traumatic in many health care institutions. Court challenges have begun to have some direct impact on the overall employment practices in many hospitals. The erosion of the "at-will" doctrine is of concern to health care management for the following reasons:

- The cost associated with each challenge or court case. A number of attorneys will take wrongful discharge cases on a contingency fee basis, so that a former employee has no cost to worry about. If there are no legal fees to pay, what has the employee to lose?

- The health care industry most likely will be in some form of economic downturn period for the next 10 years. In times of economic contraction, terminated employees have a tendency to want to sue. That tendency increases if there is a scarcity of health care jobs in their communities.

- If a former employee's suit is successful, the settlement dollars awarded are usually huge.

- Successful settlement of cases increases the potential for more plaintiffs to surface.

The employer's motive in discharging any "at-will" employees and the manner in which the discharge is carried out must be coordinated and reviewed by a skilled human resource person. The interest of the employer in managing the business, the interest of the employee in making a living, and the public's interest in maintaining the balance between the two all need to be seriously considered before employees are terminated for economic reasons.

What direction the health care worker will take to satisfy his concern with job security will in the final analysis depend on the importance that health care management gives to the question of health care job security. Positive employee relations, policies, and practices, as well as effective employee-centered management are the essentials for demonstrating to employees that they do not need a union. The NLRA specifically provides that employees have the right to refrain from joining the union. Such a choice will almost always result from employees' feeling toward upper management or their immediate supervisors and from their sense that management is dealing fairly with them not only on wages, benefits, and work conditions, but also in matters of supervision, participation, open and honest communication, reductions in labor complement, economics, and job security.

First-line supervisors will continue to bear the brunt of employee relations responsibility and problems; as discussed in the next chapter, they are the foundation of sound labor practice. Upper management's responsibility will be to respond if it wishes its facility to remain nonunion.

ENDNOTES

1.   *Taft-Hartley Amendments: Implications for the Health Care Field.* Chicago: American Hospital Association, 1975.

2.   Dennis R. Kobs, *A Guide to Employer Employee Relations.* St. Louis: Catholic Hospital Association, 1974.

3.   "The Erosion of the Termination At-Will Doctrine: Or--'Who Says I Can't Fire Them?'" Bulletin #36, Rockville, MD: Aspen Systems Corp., 1981.

CHAPTER 3

Positive Supervisory Practices to Maintain Non-union Status in a Health Care Facility

SUPERVISION AND PARTNERSHIP

Sound labor practices begin and end with the front-line supervisor. Douglas McGregor provides us with a solid analysis of strict versus lenient supervision.[1] He suggests that there are two major parts in the leadership process, both important in establishing and maintaining effective employee relation practices: Supervisors must have a warm, genuine human concern for the well-being of subordinates and, at the same time, must require and maintain a high standard of performance. Supervisors, he says, must be fair but firm with subordinates. If supervisors do not require strict standards of performance, then both performance and respect will tend to degenerate. If the supervisor is too wishy-washy, he or she cannot command the proper respect. Most importantly, these two behavior patterns must co-exist. If we are fair but not firm enough, we lose control of the group.[2]

Aside from the high-stress element always prevalent in health care employment, there are other problems unique to the supervision of health care employees. The first is that the work performed in a health care facility is greatly specialized and highly interactional. Also, there is an extensive division and diversity of education, background, and training among employees in health care facilities.

Most important, almost every person working in a health care facility depends upon some other employee for the successful completion of his/her performance. An example is the physician who needs a specimen analyzed. In order for the physician to confirm a diagnosis and properly prescribe for a patient, it is necessary that

- the unit secretary process the requisition

- the laboratory supervisor assign a technician to obtain the specimen

- the laboratory technologist conduct the appropriate tests and record findings

- the laboratory secretary communicate the findings to the patient's unit secretary

- the registered nurse convey the results to the physician and, possibly, depending on the findings, to pharmacy, radiology, occupational therapy, physical therapy, dietary, etc.

The health care supervisor frequently experiences pressure not only from upper management and employees, but also from the medical staff who are neither management nor employees but private practitioners with privileges to use the facility for their patients.

Though supervision is often referred to as a process, the steps in the procedure of supervision in a health care facility are seldom identified. Too often those who are in the role of supervisory management are themselves unaware of what is expected of them as supervisors and therefore fail to function effectively in the role.

It should be kept in mind by the supervisory manager that the basic authority and thus responsibility for the operation of a work unit has been vested through delegation in the supervisor. Therefore, whatever exists in that work unit has either been caused to exist or is permitted to exist by the supervisor. If a worker's performance is poor, the supervisor has either caused it, permitted it to remain, or both. If, on the other hand, the performance is good, this same principle will apply--the supervisor has either caused it or has permitted it.

Supervisors have the opportunity, therefore, either to permit what happens, to respond to what others make happen, or to cause what happens by their own determination and initiative. Supervisors can delegate away their authority but not their responsibility. Delegation should only create a partnership for responding to the original responsibility.

New trends in labor relations have given subordinates a right to a voice in their own destiny and legal means to exercise that right. As a result, new supervisory styles create opportunities for the employees to become involved in planning, problem solving, and decision making.

Although management may sometimes presume that it has a unique interest in the corporate process, employees also feel they have a vested interest in the well-being of the corporation.

There is a balance of power between the workforce and management. Although partially a product of legislation, this balance has become a matter of social expectation. For example, the employee no longer need be the victim of the physical surroundings but can be a voice in the determination of a safe work environment. Under the National Labor Relations Act, that same employee can also have a voice in wages and hours, the type and extent of supervision given, staffing patterns, workload distribution, performance standards, training and continuing education, and so on. Other laws give the employee a voice in self-protection from discrimination, rights to advancement, promotion, equal pay, and even rights to avoid conflict-of-conscience situations.

Based on the simple principle that one tends to resist and resent that which is imposed but tends to commit to and be motivated by that which is proposed, it would appear that supervisors have a greater opportunity to succeed by creating a team relationship with the employee. In such a relationship, supervisors would seek employees' advice, ask for their recommendations, and eventually make them part of the solution process rather than a continuance of the problem. The melding of management and labor by common interest, working through common means to fulfill common objectives, can create a true sense of teamwork.

A team wins together or loses together; a team is not composed of some winners and some losers. Teamwork is one important means of minimizing the eventual obstructionism of separate interest pursuits and the split of management and labor groups destined for confrontation. The extent to which employees enjoy a general sense of security in the employment situation, the extent to which they have respect for and confidence in management, and the extent to which they have a sense of identity, recognition and dignity within the organization will determine the extent to which the sense of a true team relationship is possible. When employees are insecure, lack respect for and confidence in management, or do not feel their identity is recognized by dignity, they have the choice to quit and seek satisfaction elsewhere or to remain and find a new means other than through management to gain that to which they feel entitled. It is not the management that votes union or no union in an NLRB election, but the employees.

SUPERVISORY AND OPERATIONAL RECOMMENDATIONS

It is only natural for each of us to attempt to increase our assets and decrease our liabilities. In the work situation, there is a basic desire to increase our wages, improve our benefits, add to our leisure time, undertake new avenues of training and continuing education, increase the social satisfactions from work, and seek the incentives and rewards of advancement and promotion. At the same time, it is equally natural to minimize or reduce what is expected of us, reduce the number of tasks or the amount of work to be performed, shorten the length of the workday or workweek, divide or share responsibilities with fellow workers, or make work easier by obtaining better tools, supplies, facilities, and so on.

EFFECTIVE SUPERVISORY PRACTICES

Given these concerns and the foregoing thoughts, several preliminary recommendations are possible. These recommendations are aimed not so much at action but at a sound philosophy of supervision that should precede implementation of more specific recommendations discussed on page 27.

1. Administrators and managers should accept the principles of participatory management and recognize that employees can be partners in solving problems. This may be accomplished in a formal organization or through ad hoc committee structures.

2. Where employee and management groups are working on morale issues, it is strongly suggested that specific objectives for such group activity be established as a means of both guiding the deliberations of the group and evaluating the end product. Presentation of specific objectives offers a method of maintaining administrative control while actually helping rather than hindering the process of group voice and decision-making.

3. As solutions and decisions are proposed to reduce or resolve current problems, it is crucial that the administration be specific in assigning the authority for the implementation of any action program to a specific person, department, or group. Along with designating the authority, the administration should identify a target date when accountability will be required.

4. To maintain employee confidence and administrative credibility on basic operational issues, it is essential to have continuous communication in the form of reports to subordinate levels of management and to the employees on investigations, projects, assignment of actions, and the success of problem reduction. Knowledge of results (KOR) is deemed to be the most essential factor in the learning process, and time has indicated that it is equally essential in building morale and achieving a sense of community. Delays in the achievement of any project can be expected. Reports are not appreciated, however, if all that is made known is the fact that there have been no results.

   A simple one- or two-page memo once or twice a week can reinforce the communication process. It may be titled simply "Administrative Update," "Administrative Action Line," or "People, Projects, and Progress." It should be appropriately numbered and dated, have identifying topics in the left margin, and include brief paragraph descriptions of status and achievement reports. This becomes a simple, ongoing process of vital communication. Second, it serves as a means of exercising accountability over the persons, groups, and/or departments assigned specific authority to work out solutions to identified problems. To some extent it redirects criticism and even anger from the administration to others who now have the responsibility to provide the remedies that will achieve operational improvement.

Viewing these preliminary recommendations more as a style or approach, it is important now to direct attention to some of the operational practices that would seem most appropriate in attempting to remedy or at least reduce general problems within the health care facility.

SPECIFIC OPERATIONAL PRACTICES

Staffing Pattern Control and Workload Distribution

One of the most difficult questions for a supervisor to answer is the exact number of workers required to meet the work requirements of a particular area of the operation. There is always the concern of the employee who feels pushed, rushed, pressured, overworked, or even exploited. This is in contrast to the concerns of management that an employee is underproductive, that labor costs consume too much of the operating income, that current demands for increased staffing are not legitimate based on workload requirements in light of past performance levels and staffing patterns, and so on. There are a number of unfortunate factors that further complicate the staffing question.

- **Lack of work control.** Supervisors have done little to appropriately plan, design, describe, analyze, and control work. It is the type of work, its frequency and quantity, the time the work must be performed, and the place where it must be done that eventually define requirements for the type of workforce, the number of workers, when the workers must be available, and where they must be assigned. In the absence of controlled work, there is no control of staffing.

- **Misconceptions about staffing.** Staffing tends to be viewed as the number of bodies for the available productive hours--a point of view shared by supervisors and workers. This unfortunately denies the supervisor four other essential control aspects of the final staffing:

  1. There can be ample working bodies or productive hours available, but the incumbent staff lacks appropriate knowledge, skills, or general qualifications to perform what must be performed. The result is that at the end of a given work period, work has not been completed, leading to the belief that more staff members are needed.

  2. There may be an ample number of competent workers, but they have been assigned inappropriate work to perform. The nurse pursues clerical functions as the nurse's aide pursues housekeeping

functions, for example. By the end of the day, there may still be duties to be performed by the nurse and nurse's aide, again prompting the conclusion that there is a staff shortage when the problem, in fact, is inappropriate assignment or pursuit of work.

3. An ample number of capable workers performing the right functions could be using inappropriate, obsolete, or ineffective techniques, procedures, and methods. Therefore, what might otherwise be accomplished in 10 minutes could require 20; the time is spent chasing supply items rather than performing the task. This results in leftover work at the end of the work period, which is easily taken as a sign of too few workers rather than too little efficiency.

4. Finally, it is possible to have an appropriate number of qualified and competent workers performing the right activities int he right way, but the workers themselves are undermotivated and have little inclination to perform effectively. Once again the work is not completed in the assigned work time, giving the appearance that more workers are needed to get the work done.

Essentially, these thoughts suggest that supervisors should view obtaining more workers not as a first step but as a last step, giving first effort to an evaluation of motivation, work techniques, procedures and methods, appropriate work distribution, and the determination of appropriate factors in competency for performance. Even one additional worker should be viewed as the absolute last resort.

Obviously, these are difficult evaluations to make. Thee is a need to determine what the individual worker is doing; develop position descriptions; analyze each task in terms of purpose, procedure, method, and performance standards; extract performance requirements from such work information, compare performance requirements with competency inventories of incumbents; pursue a formal work-distribution project; and attempt to involve the worker in a sufficient number of work decisions to capture interest and provide motivation.

There are natural byproducts of the above steps that will be valuable in overcoming any concerns of the employee that job descriptions are missing or perhaps are incomplete, inaccurate, or irrelevant in terms of duties actually required or performed. Detailed task analyses will provide appropriate training aids, including procedures, methods, and performance standards. Better criteria for selection through improved performance requirements will ensure a better matching of future workers to the job, minimizing insecurity and other problems relating to inadequate and incompetent performance.

Communication and the Right to Relate

Prudent supervisors should manage as though a militant union is outside--because it is. From now on, the health care industry can expect that some dissatisfied group of employees might either initiate or respond to organized labor as a representative for the purpose of resolving employee-employer relationship problems. Viewing the collective bargaining process as a means rather than as an objective, it becomes obvious that the only contributing factor that this process provides is a basis for communication. Since the National Labor Relations Act simply provides by law a structural framework so that management and the workforce can relate to each other in "good faith," it seems important to determine alternative means of providing both the communication process and the exercise of mutual good faith.

When one party speaks or writes, there is an expectation that the other party will listen or read--actually focus on what the ear has heard or the eye has observed. Part of the problem, it seems, is notifying the other party that an attempted exchange of an idea is about to occur.

The simple X plus Y equals Z formula applied to labor relations is reduced to doing right voluntarily (the X) plus getting credit for it (the Y) which should equal realistic employee-employer relationships (the Z). Even for supervisors who may be fully effective in understanding employee needs, responding to them, and assisting employees in responding to the needs of supervisors, there is still the absolute necessity to take time to inform the employees in such a way that they understand, accept, or give credit for what has been accomplished. This will result in a realistic relationship.

The communication process is necessary to assist in achieving the right relationship--and, at the same time, the establishment of the right relationship becomes vital to the process of communication. Somewhere that circle must be penetrated with an action system.

There is value in following the simple process of checking up on one's communication effectiveness. Whether in the one-to-one situation, in small group conferences, or through written media, it is wise to occasionally evaluate the effort by asking for the opinion of the target of your communication.

One other simple thought is worth remembering: The complexity of attempting to achieve effective communication justifies attempting to minimize communication needs. Therefore, the involvement of employees as team members or partners with supervisors in the problem-solving and decision-making processes achieves a sense not only of commitment to the outcome but also of communication.

Supervisory Human Relations Training

The preschool child sitting before a television learns the importance of "please" and "thank you." For some reason, as adults and as supervisors we seem to ignore these simple human relations expressions. Employees feel that they are told, not asked, to perform, and that there is little appreciation expressed. There is a sense of exploitation rather than recognition of the dignity of the individual person.

Having lived through the decade of the 1960s, the younger generation in particular has been exposed to equal rights, civil rights, women's rights, equal employment opportunity rights, and so on. The importance of the individual is emphasized in the 1199 National Union Hospital and Health Care Employees campaign slogan "I am somebody." The employee wants to be identified in his own right and recognized for his own dignity. There is a highly sensitive reaction to cases of partiality, favoritism, or open discrimination, and most workers abhor sexism and racism.

The lack of expressed appreciation, the failure to seek employee advice, the failure to follow employee recommendations, and incidences of partiality and favoritism can lead to serious breakdowns in the fundamental human relationship between supervisors and employees. The emphasis should be on a sincere, concerned, and caring relationship between management and its workforce--in the context, of course, of maintenance of discipline and respect and the adherence to performance standards and overall policies.

The use of the terms "please" and "thank you" by supervisors would seem to be an important starting point. The word "please" does not rule against an expected response and does not rule out firmness. It is simply a change in the manner of approach. The response of "thank you" simply reflects what some research has indicated--that an employee expects more than a monetary return for his effort. The term "thank you" contains within it a sense of recognition and appreciation, both of which are important.

It is important that supervisors view each employee as a prospective friend. A person makes friends one at a time and not by group action. This means that mutual understanding, trust, respect, and confidence are vital. At the same time, supervisors must maintain their own dignity and status in the organization and must be respected. The basic virtues of openness, honesty, truth-seeking, freedom-building, and community achievement of mutual respect all have a particular place in the relationship between supervisors and the workforce.

The employment situation today is based upon satisfactory workers (meaning the fulfillment of the supervisor's needs) and satisfied workers (meaning the fulfillment of the employee's needs). When an employee is no longer satisfactory, the appropriate supervisor must solve the problem through training, counseling, discipline, or discharge. When an employee is no longer satisfied, he or she has a variety of resources by which to solve the alleged problem. The employee may confront the situation personally with the supervisor, lean upon some appropriate government agency, or respond to or initiate contact with organized labor or the organized professional associations to pursue voluntary collective bargaining.

It is important to keep in mind, then, that the personal relationship between each employee and his or her immediate supervisor, coupled with the degree to which the employee feels that the supervisor who is now a friend is supported by higher management, will provide the resources through which the employee can voice concerns. The employee who enjoys a realistic sense of security coupled with a sense of confidence in management in an environment of productive and satisfied human relationships is not the employee who will turn to an outside third party as a representative. The burden to prevent outside representation rests with supervisors; the choice rests with the worker.

ENDNOTES

1.   McGregor, Douglas, *The Human Side of Enterprise*. New York: McGraw-Hill Book Co., Inc., 1959.

2.   Thomas R. O'Donovan, Ph.D., *Effective Supervision Requires Leadership. Hospital Organization and Management*, St Louis: Catholic Hospital Association, 1972.

CHAPTER 4
The Substance of Labor Relations: Critical Factors

When there are realistic feelings of security, when there is confidence in management, a feeling of supportive relationships, and if there exists a significant system for rewarding good work within the employment context, the results are strong and positive employee-management relations. The reverse situation is equally true. The challenge to management, therefore, is to find means by which to know the status of these factors in the employees' minds and then to pursue constructive action to turn negative views into positive and substantive views.

When the above factors are not present, a worker will often seek third party intervention. This might be a claim with the Occupational Safety and Health Review Commission of unsafe working conditions. There may be a claim with the Human Rights Commission through which the support of the Equal Employment Opportunity Commission can be gained if the employee feels that there are discriminatory or unfair relationships. The lack of confidence that there is equal pay for equal work regardless of sex provides opportunity to file a claim with the Department of Labor for investigation and support in legal actions to gain equity. General dissatisfaction with one's supervisor or management in general or with wages, hours, or working conditions could draw the attention of an organizer for a labor union or a professional association who could then pursue legal support for intervention through the National Labor Relations Board.

While these are avenues by which an employee can seek to rectify what is viewed as an inappropriate condition for employment, some employees would simply quit and seek to find their sense of satisfaction elsewhere. There are always those, however, who remain firmly entrenched in their jobs, where they become potential sources of turmoil as they seek to contaminate other employees with their frustrations, tensions, and dissatisfactions.

The organizer for a labor union has been schooled in techniques to give employees a strong sense of insecurity--to disrupt productive and positive relationships within the organization, destroy employees' sense of confidence in management, and point out the insignificance or lack of reward employees derive through employment. This suggests that even when management attempts to develop and preserve these important factors, there is still the risk that counterefforts could be more productive, particularly as society moves toward more liberal viewpoints of rights and establishes new and different expectations from employers.

Each of these factors has many facets that may present either opportunities for constructive development or risks of deterioration. Some of these facts are:

33

- **Security.** The employee is first concerned over the security of the job--will it last? A high unemployment rate may stimulate a high level of insecurity despite the fact that the health care field has demonstrated job stability.

  Employees get a sense of security from both their paychecks and their benefits. Sick leave obviously gives a sense of economic security in the event the employee falls ill and is unable to work. Workers' Compensation provides security in the event of a job injury, accident or occupational disease. The retirement pension offers security for one's senior years. A life insurance benefit offers the peace of mind that one's family may be secure. Good health and hospitalization benefits provide the security of paying the cost of health care services without jeopardizing one's standard of living or lifestyle.

  There is also the security of capable management, responsive to one's needs and supportive on the job. Adequate orientation, job training and continuing education provide security against obsolescence and incompetency deficiencies. Quite simply, nearly everything management does, it can do so as to enhance employee security or to ignore and even disturb it. It is therefore vital that management do what it can to relate its efforts to employee security. The employee who relies solely on the quality of his own performance or the shortage of qualified labor in the local market for his sense of security, takes security out from under the control of management and leaves management the victim of outside influences that might negate security.

- **Confidence in management.** Management can be a force for either good or evil. When it is responsive to the needs and desires of the employees, it is viewed as a force for good. When employees view management as a force of positive concern, they tend to give not only their confidence but also their trust and eventually their loyalty, dedication, and commitment to management and what management fosters. This is especially important in these times of persistent social and political pressures on the health care industry in general and managers in particular. Confidence emerges when employees believe in management's integrity and dependability to respond to changing needs with appropriate actions and sensitivity. Employees who lack a sense of confidence in management will tend to find some other source in which to place that confidence--a senior worker, organized labor, the federal government or even another employer.

- **A sense of supportive relationships.** People do not cease to be social beings when they enter the workplace. Relationships between co-workers tend to develop quite naturally, but good relationships between employees and supervisors are also of great importance. They are professional friendships, one-to-one and face-to-face. When the employees are sensitive and the supervisors are caring, their relationships can eliminate the "we and they" syndrome between workers and management.

Too often, however, supervisors go overboard in their efforts to avoid acting "superior." When employees are led to think of their immediate supervisors as peer workers and higher management as some distant "they," the necessary professional distinctions are blurred.

Supervisors should instead concentrate on establishing their credibility, integrity, and dependability. Credible supervisors will gain employee confidence. Then, by demonstrating--through action at least as much as through words--their integrity and dependability, they will be able to establish appropriate relationships with the employees. Instead of "we" and "they," there will be a sense of common purpose and a recognition of each person's role in working toward that purpose.

- **A sense of significance or reward.** Compensation is not always limited to the wages and benefits earned through productive performance. The significance of one's work, the reputation of the employer, or the simple feeling of being appreciated can often provide that essential sense of reward that is as important as cash compensation.

  It is important, however, to recognize that most people do not live to work--they work in order to live, and the means to that living are wages and benefits. These forms of compensation, therefore, must be considered vital factors in the employee-management relationship--but by themselves they cannot develop and sustain overall satisfaction. Praise, recognition, respect for individual dignity, a simple "thank you" from time to time all add to this sense of significance and reward. Employees' basic social and psychological needs can be as important as their economic needs.

When personalities, policies, practices, and procedures twist the employment conditions so that the foregoing factors are uncertain or negative, the possibility of any type of effective employee-management relationship is diminished, if not destroyed. Continued neglect of appropriate actions to overcome such problems can and often does lead to third-party intervention. The unsatisfied employee has three alternatives. First, the employee can simply grin and bear it, tolerating the conditions in the belief that there are no other alternatives. Second, the employee can quit and seek employment elsewhere, hoping to find that these primary factors and the many related issues are positive, and thus find satisfaction. Finally, the employee has the option of seeking a union and collective bargaining or the intervention of federal investigative agencies to give either social and economic leverage or legal support in rectifying those conditions that the employee views as inappropriate.

Management's foreknowledge of the employee view affords the opportunity to pursue corrective action or the chance to reinform the employee of the management view. There must be common understanding before there can be acceptance. When management fails to initiate actions that will lead to improved employee-management relations, it can only be viewed as management's fault when the employee is no longer an advocate for management's position. Despite the variety of federal controls through labor legislation, management still remains the means to either avoid or overcome an adversary relationship.

CHAPTER 5

Confrontation, Conflict, or Collaboration and Cooperation?

The era of the 1960s is now referred to as the "age of rights," the "Great Society." The view then was that "life can be changed." In the 1970s, the emphasis was on "doubt." Institutions were breaking down; they were top heavy and cumbersome. The social maxim of the 70s was "everybody for himself." The epoch of the 1980s focuses on the salient psychological forces that depict the problems in the management of people.

Thus, the sociology from 1960s to the 1980s has resulted in new pressures for the democratization of management practices and the recognition of the individual worker as a partner in the employee-employer relationship. Neither the employee nor the employer wants dependency, but realistically neither can sustain an independent position. What is possible and now necessary is recognition of an interdependent relationship. The federal labor laws involving the health care field--beginning in the mid-60s with the Fair Labor Standards Act Amendment, the Occupational Safety and Health Act, the Civil Rights Act and subsequent guidelines of the Equal Employment Opportunity Commission, through the passage in 1974 of the National Labor Relations Act as amended for health care facilities--have each given the employee a unique source of power by bringing the support of the federal system to rectify those conditions that may violate the employees' economic rights, their rights for a safe and hazard-free work environment, their social rights, or their rights to confront management to negotiate changes in their wages, hours or working conditions. The balance of power is real.

Sensitive supervisors now recognize that employees are more than bodies hired to perform specific tasks. They are specialists in understanding their own jobs, supervisors, and work conditions. They understand their own needs and objectives better than anyone else. They come to the job complete with reason and emotion that determine how they think and feel about the physical, social, psychological, moral, economic, and managerial environments in which they must work. They want their own identities. They want to be recognized, to be heard, and to have a voice in the decision-making process that affects their destinies. As a result, what employees think and feel becomes a real factor in the employee-employer relationship and in the eventual acceptance or rejection of the policies and practices established by management for that relationship.

If an employee thinks there is a problem, then there is. If the problem exists in fact, then management must, through corrective action, remedy the situation. On the other hand, if there is no problem in fact, there is the need for corrective communication so that the employee will understand the situation from the same point of view as it is understood by management.

As we wrote in an earlier work, "Understanding how the employee views the various managerial practices becomes an absolute necessity for enlightened management to plan appropriately that which must be done to maintain a cooperative workforce that is both satisfied and satisfactory."[1] Management as the leadership of the operation can no longer permit what happens to happen. Management cannot be in control if it merely increases its sensitivity and perception of what is happening in order to respond to it. What is needed is a causative force determining what must occur for the mutual benefit of all concerned and executing the appropriate actions to ensure that what must happen does in fact happen.

According to Keith Davis, "There is a difference in the way management approaches people to motivate them. If the approach emphasizes rewards--economic or otherwise--for the followers, the manager is using positive leadership. If the emphasis is on penalties--the manager is viewed as applying negative leadership."[2] This reasoning applies also to the individual supervisory styles--employee-oriented and production-oriented. The employee-oriented supervisor (management) is compassionate and respects the rights and dignity of workers. The production-oriented supervisor (management) doesn't mind sending signals out to the employee that the institution comes first and all else is secondary. The two styles do not need to be at opposite ends of the spectrum. Management can use both in varying degrees. Likewise, it is possible to have a working combination of management philosophies such as paternal, accommodating, cooperative, autocratic, and participatory each working productively for both the institution and the employees. Health care employees in their work environment seek more than a paycheck. It is acknowledged that, like other workers, health care employees work to satisfy physical needs; but when the fundamental needs of life such as food, clothing, and shelter are met, health care workers often expect more out of the work relationship than do workers in other industries.

Health care facilities are sociological organizations made up of doctors, nurses, technologists, aides, various levels and types of professionals, tradespeople, administrative personnel, clerks and service workers. This sociological mix lends itself to establishing conflict within the institution. Differences of opinion, jealousy, "turfism," and egotism are the most prevalent causes of confrontation and conflict in health care facilities.

In the nursing homes and/or long-term care facilities there is a slight modification of the confrontation and conflict formula. In these facilities the nurse aides are a major component of the labor complement. They perform work of the highest order, caring continuously for the multiple needs of their elderly patients, frequently under very adverse conditions. These long-term care nurse aides are expected to be the custodians of terminal cases, and as such bear particularly heavy burdens. Yet they occupy no prestigious position within the sociological status of the health care institution.

It is imperative that health care management analyze and seek to meet the needs of all its employees, category by category. If it is determined that the employees' basic physical needs are being met equitably and fairly, then management must seek to develop a plan to meet the other needs such as safety, security, a feeling of belonging, appreciation, self-esteem, and finally self-actualization[3] for all sociological levels within the institution.

ENDNOTES

1.   Rene Laliberty and W. I. Christopher, *Enhancing Productivity in Health Care Facilities.* Owings Mills, MD: National Health Publishing, 1984.

2.   Keith Davis, Ph.D., *Human Relations at Work--The Dynamics of Organizational Behavior.* New York: McGraw-Hill, 1967.

3.   A. H. Maslow's theory of need priority based upon physiology, safety and security, middle order and higher order. "A Theory of Human Motivation," *Psychological Review.* New York: Harper & Row, Inc., 1954.

CHAPTER 6

The Governing Board: Last Step in Internal Control for a Health Care Facility Labor Relations Program

Despite assumptions to the contrary, health care trustees and/or directors are not all appointed as equals. All do not have common knowledge and experience in administration and its various subdivisions. Each member of the governing board thus has a different level of understanding of his function, administration's function, and the significance of the operation of the health care facility. This means that new appointees, and often the established directors, need intensive orientation if there is to be effective decision-making.

The governing board's greatest responsibility is patient care. Their second greatest responsibility is personnel. It is the work performed by personnel that contributes to the achievement of patient care. The quality of that performance and the wisdom by which the work was designed determine the effectiveness of the work. The resources used by employees determine the efficiency and resultant cost of that work.

The greatest external pressures on governing boards tend to center on social and political reaction to the health care delivery system. The main internal problems are many. The directors tend to focus on financial management in response to pressures for cost containment. To keep pace with code modification and continually changing standards for patient safety they direct most of their attention almost exclusively toward facilities, organizational structure, and product line management. They also focus on whether or not the health care facility is properly equipped to keep pace with the changing medical field as it impacts on an evolving health care delivery system.

The mutual dependence of the physician and the health care facility requires attention to professional relations. The political arena and its intended control over health care operations demand that attention also be directed to a wide range of investigating and planning agencies. The net result would seem to be that there is too little time remaining to devote appropriate attention to human resource matters. A quick examination of the minutes of the preceding year of governing board meetings will indicate the frequency and the intensity with which the board has reviewed and acted upon human resource issues.

ESTABLISHING THE RIGHT OF THE GOVERNING BOARD TO KNOW

One might wonder why there is any question of the governing board's right to know what is occurring in the personnel program when the board has both ultimate authority and ultimate responsibility. The fact of the matter is that the right to know is not merely a respect for that authority or an obedience, but a necessity if the governing board is to carry out its role and function in terms of current concepts of health care administration. There are several views therefore that need examination.

- **Democratized authority.** The historical basis of health care administration has emerged from three primary sources: religion, medicine, and the military, all three of which have tended in the past to be authoritarian. During the 1960s the inherent rights and dignity of the individual gained recognition. When transferred to business situations, this concept caused changes in management style from authoritarianism to a more democratized form. Democratization was translated operationally as a system of participative management. Just as democracy separates the judicial, executive, and legislative functions, so these three subfactors of management had to be separated for participative management within the facility. In terms of the facility as a whole, the governing board must judge, the chief executive officer and management team must execute, and the technical directors of key disciplines must legislate. This establishes a basis for accountability.

  To legislate is to recommend. To execute is to accept or reject that which is recommended and to implement that which is accepted. To judge is to determine standards that are set arbitrarily by authority and that must be used as a basis of measuring or evaluating the norms created by organizational behavior. Measurement, which is quantitative, and evaluation, which is qualitative, lead to a judgment as to whether the norm is above, at, or below the standard that provides the opportunity for the exercise of corrective action or control. To judge effectively, the governing board has not only the right but also the obligation to know what is occurring within the organization in order that appropriate judgments can be rendered and control maintained.

- **Knowledge as opportunity.** By knowing what is occurring within the organization, the governing board has an opportunity to influence the organization--for example, to protect the operation through objective evaluation and control. Knowledge allows the board to participate through the exercise of corrective action--to propose changes in operational practice--and also through praise where it is due. The board may pursue a particular issue or prod in areas where there has been little movement. In brief, the knowledge of what is occurring enables the board to participate actively in the operation of the health care facility without interfering with the operators.

- **Human resource systems.** Human resource administration is an integral part of and an extension of basic administration. With the new emphasis on cost containment, it is necessary to establish systems for resource management. Collective administration must allocate resources, while technical directors or heads of major disciplines must provide systems to utilize resources in the most effective and efficient manner consistent with achieving the desired results. First-line supervisors must apply the resources to the workers' performance to ensure those results. Since human resource administration seeks to integrate work and worker, knowledge of what is occurring within the personnel program is vital to the ultimate responsibility of the governing board--quality patient care. Human resource administration is the design of a personnel program, in contrast to personnel management, which is the implementation of that program. Administration is the responsibility of the administrator delegated to the human resource director. Personnel management is the responsibility of the supervisor.

Although there are other reasons that justify the governing board's right to know, these three fundamental concepts establish the basis for the board's interest in knowing what is occurring in the personnel program.

SPECIFIC PERSONNEL ADMINISTRATION INFORMATION THAT THE GOVERNING BOARD SHOULD KNOW

A listing of the specifics of the personnel program can serve as a summary for a comprehensive personnel program. Because the personnel program affects every other aspect of the operation--patient care, medical staff satisfaction, community relations, cost of care, and so on--a simple review of its essential concerns could aid directors. These specific areas of concern are as follows:

- **Analyzing the work.** Since the work specifies resources and determines final costs as well as the quality of the end product of performance, there is a need to know how work is controlled. Is there a means of identifying or determining what each individual worker does? Are there appropriate methods for distributing work to the appropriate competency level? Do job descriptions exist that accurately reflect what the worker does? Have tasks been analyzed so there is appropriate understanding of purpose, procedure, method, and performance standards? Since the type of work and the amount of work determines the number and type of personnel required, is there emphasis on work simplification and methods improvement in order to enhance the performance of necessary work with minimal use of personnel? Is there effort to use automation to replace labor?

- **More than numbers.** Staffing is not merely dividing a number of employees. Each employee must be appropriately competent, must be effectively deployed or assigned the right tasks to perform, must be utilizing efficient procedures and methods, and must be adequately motivated. All too often criticism of staffing is limited to complaints of understaffing, when in reality the number of employees may be adequate but the competency level is not. When an employee is permitted to do work other than that which is appropriate for the level of competency, there is not only an increase in cost for the performance of that work, but also a question as to who performs the work appropriate to that employee. The use of obsolete or inefficient procedures and methods may, in fact, prolong the time required to perform work, thus placing pressure on the performer, which results in a feeling of understaffing. Obviously, the lack of motivation can simply result in a lack of productivity and a demand for more personnel to accomplish the work that must be performed.

The board should know to what extent is there concern over factors other than the simple count of different types of personnel? What is the basis for determining the types of employees who must be hired and how many must be on duty? How is an individual employee utilized and what is the productivity of the employees individually and collectively?

The employment process reaches out into the community to recruit appropriate applicants for the workforce. Applicants must be carefully screened and eventually selected, placed, oriented, trained, directed, counseled, disciplined, and perhaps--when not performing satisfactorily-- terminated. This employment process must meet legal conditions as well as provide for operational human relations.

The governing board must understand the location of the facility's labor market and the expectations of both quantity and quality of applicants that might be forthcoming from that market. Whereas the maid, the diet aide, the clerk or the mechanic might reflect the local labor market, the nurse, the therapist, the technologist, or the department director may, in fact, reflect a regional or even a national labor market. This may call for different short-term and long-term recruitment activities, and also different wages and benefits to attract those in that labor market potentially desired by the facility. Several questions arise: What is the search process? Do performance requirements exist? And, if so, are they legal and job-validated? Employment is a mutual consideration.

Once the personnel office effectively screens applicants so no one not potentially qualified enters the workforce, who selects that one employee who is hired? Does that individual have the qualifications to conduct such a selection process? Do selectees meet immediate requirements for performance and the potential requirements for growth, advancement, and upward mobility?

Placing an employee in the organization is no longer a matter of signing him in and escorting him to the site of work. It is a systematic process of orientation and introducing him to the facility, the department, and the job, acquainting him with the environment and the factors that will be utilized in the performance of work.

All employees require training since training is the application of one's competency to the tasks as they are to be performed in that institution. Who trains--and how is training evaluated? Continuing education is the process of assisting the employee to acquire new levels of competency for growth, advancement, and ultimate promotion. How is continuing education established? Who attends? How are they evaluated? What are the positive consequences resulting to the organization from this expense and effort? Who counsels the employee, and is there adequate competency to perform this function? Similarly, who maintains discipline? How is it done? Is it consistent with laws on nondiscrimination and employee rights? What are the conditions that may lead to discharge, and how are employee rights protected in such circumstances? How is a deserving employee who must terminate employment recognized, and are such employee's rights honored?

- **Establishing wages and benefits.** Since payroll and employee benefits constitute the major factor in any operating budget, there is need to know the basis on which wages are determined and payroll dollars are distributed. Has there been job evaluation resulting in job classification and a basis for internal equity in the distribution of payroll dollars? Are there adequate wage and benefit surveys or continuing monitoring of the labor market? Are wages viewed essentially as an investment for which a return is expected, or simply as one more expense? Are there adequate means appropriately utilized that justify the wages paid based on the performance received?

What are the signs of employee confidence in the overall wage system? What is the labor turnover rate in contrast to the stability rate? To what extent is the facility able to recruit and hire the quantity and quality of employees necessary to perform essential work? Is there supporting wage policy that recognizes pay for performance, longevity, special assignment, temporary assignment to higher positions, overtime, call pay, report pay, and a host of other facets of a comprehensive wage policy? What are the philosophy and the objectives that support the overall wage program?

As a principle to which, of course, there are exceptions, one recruits with wages but retains with benefits. To what extent is the full economic package of benefits consistent with competitors for the facility's employees? Are there effective means by which the facility continually communicates to the employee the actual or real value of the benefits in addition to the cash wage received, so that there is appropriate understanding and acceptance of the full wage, not merely the paycheck?

- **Rules and policies.** With work under control, an effective process to place employees on the job, and a meaningful wage system to compensate the employee, it is important to establish the general umbrella of rules, regulations, and policies that assure a meaningful relationship of employee to employee and employees to management.

  There is need for assurance that the facility's policies are fully understood and implemented. In what areas are there rights for department directors or supervisors to establish departmental or work unit policies? To what extent can such departmental or unit policies modify--by either a more liberal or a more conservative position--the policies of the institution? Are policies in compliance with a variety of governmental or accrediting regulations? Are policies consistently interpreted and enforced? Are there appropriate procedures for implementation of the policy? Are terms defined and exceptions identified?

  Do policies provide for means of reward or punishment as the individual requires? Are they reviewed and revised as necessary? Have they been approved by the appropriate board? Are personnel policies appropriately published and distributed to the employees with realistic orientation to assure understanding? Are supervisors given additional support to allow them to interpret and enforce the policy as intended? Where appropriate, are policies--such as those regarding grievances--modified to recognize the differences in the roles of employees, supervisors, and managers?

- **Effective communications.** Human relations are best established and maintained by effective means of communication. Until there is communication, there cannot be a relationship. It is therefore important for the governing board to understand the facility's systems for effective vertical and lateral communication. Is there appropriate recognition of the value of two-way communication or dialogue that can lead to decisions and then actions, which make employees party to the communicating process and final results? Is there appropriate understanding of what should be communicated to whom, by whom, and through what means? Is the timing of a communication appropriate to the communication itself? Is the communication process simply a flow of information or is it a true exchange of ideas that enhances the operation? Is communication intended to achieve understanding that leads to acceptance, participation, or recommendation--so that each communication has a consequence?

- **Levels of management.** In recognition of an old concept that management is not to work and the workers are not to manage--a concept that is not in conflict with properly executed participative management--questions must be raised as to what each level of management is expected to do. There are distinctions between the first-line supervisor, the middle manager or department director, and the administrative staff. To what extent have the jobs been clarified and described? Are there appropriate performance requirements used in the selection or promotion of employees to management positions? What are the assurances that the management levels are functioning as they ought to and have the competency to function effectively? What provisions have been made for orientation, training, and continuing education of supervisory personnel? What are the criteria for performance standards, and how are management personnel evaluated? To what extent do first-line supervisors comply with the National Labor Relations checklist on supervision? Do supervisors meet the criteria for exempt status as executive personnel under the Fair Labor Standards Act?

   How are supervisory attitudes monitored? To what extent do supervisors support higher levels of management? To what extent are the relationships with working personnel consistent with the philosophy, objective, and policies of administration? How do individual supervisors influence the operation in positive directions? In a labor crisis, would the supervisor be the support that the facility needs or be part of the problem that confronts the entity?

- **Grievance systems.** Whenever two or more individuals must relate on a consistent basis, there is the risk of problems arising and eventually grievances emerging. It is therefore essential that a comprehensive personnel program provide appropriate systems for problem reduction or resolution and grievance settlements.

   What systems prevail? Are they simple to use? Do employees demonstrate confidence that the systems can be used? Who has used the systems? For what purpose--and what were the results? In light of concerns that voicing a complaint will create resentment or possible reprisal, what are the protections provided for an employee who tries to resolve problems and settle grievances? Are there assurances to the employee that

grievances are not placed in the record and considered during performance reviews? Are there means for representing employees who may
be timid or limited in education or in the communication skills?

Are current problems of limited duration or do they reflect long periods
of time without resolution? Are problems resolved as near the source of
the problem as possible? Are there means for appeal and does the appeal
system provide protection for the lower level of supervision--not necessarily providing blind support for what may have been inappropriate settlement or solution?

- **Human development.** Human development is often referred to as the
  modern concept that distinguishes real management from subordinate
  functions of directing things. What, then, is the facility's human development force, its system for growth, advancement and promotion? Are
  there adequate continuing education opportunities and growth experiences provided by which employees can acquire new competencies? Is
  there a manpower table or system by which employees can move both
  laterally and vertically in the system, dependent upon qualification and
  job opportunity? Are opportunities made known both to employees and
  to sublevels of management, so that incumbent work staff has first opportunity for advancement? Is there a sense among personnel within the
  organization that the institution is a good place to work and that employees have a good future by making a commitment to the facility?

  To what extent are the opportunities to learn situational--emanating out
  of the job itself or the environment, rather than formal systems? Are
  there systems to encourage further employee education through academic
  centers, such as a tuition reimbursement policy as an incentive? Does the
  average supervisor truly view the development of the subordinate workforce as a responsibility?

- **Relationships and rights.** It is important that the human relationships in
  the employment situation--whether between co-workers or between employees and managers--be established without favoritism, partiality, or
  discrimination. Is there a means within the health care facility by which
  an employee can get a response to an alleged infraction of human rights
  before a third party intervenes? Within the system is there appropriate
  counseling to enhance effective human relationships and, where there are
  disruptions to that relationship, are there appropriate means of discipline?
  Is the policy supporting discipline a fair and just policy, and is it exercised without favor or discrimination?

- **Appropriate participation.** Is there a true system of employee partici-
  pation--with, however, appropriate supervision so that the employees are
  not in effect attempting to run the operation? Is there true collaboration

on problem solving and decision making at the appropriate work unit level where the employee has sufficient competency to be effective? Is the employee's voice heard, and how do higher levels of management respond?

- **The personnel department and the board.** The personnel department must make many reports and complete many questionnaires, and is often subject to specific audits and assessments. To what extent is the governing board made aware of the conclusions of such audits or assessments? Is the board in accord with the information provided by the personnel administration to the various outside agencies and governmental investigatory bodies? Is the present practice consistent with board philosophy and objectives? Is the personnel office providing adequate research to investigate or to validate its operations?

- **Services for employees.** As part of any comprehensive personnel program, there may be a variety of services provided to the employee that are considered free benefits but actually constitute major functions. These may include cafeteria service for meals for employees; parking lot availability for parking; locker rooms for protection of personal effects; provision for uniforms and the appropriate laundry of same; a health center for physical examinations, annual checkups, and emergency care; and a social and recreational program. There are costs directly attributable to such services. There are benefits that are expected in employee relations as a result of such services. To what extent are these services monitored and evaluated? Are they understood, accepted, and appreciated for the value that they have to the employee? Are there services that must be provided that are not part of the system?

- **The result: confidence.** As a net result of all the foregoing items, do the employees have confidence in management? Is there a mutual sense that administration supports the interest of the employees and, in turn, the employees are responsive by supporting the programs of administration? Is there appropriate response time to problems, grievances, and recommendations? Is management visible, approachable, and credible to the employees, based on its decisions and actions?

  Does the administration "market" to the employees so that the personnel program is understood, accepted, supported and appreciated? Is there a means by which dissatisfactions on the part of employees or administration can be made known and the response realized?

Once the governing board directs its attention to many of the above items, operational practice will occasionally identify other specifics that must also be made known. The directors need to have such knowledge; therefore, the personnel director needs to respond to appropriate reports. From the point of view of the personnel director, a knowledgeable governing board is not an interference, but rather a unique source of support and approval for future modifications that must be made in the personnel program to keep pace with changing styles of management and expectations of the workforce.

Administration, which includes the governing board, must allocate resources appropriate to the work that must be performed in order to fulfill the mission of the institution. As it benefits from awareness of the various aspects of the program that enhances the utilization of the human resource in the organization, the board will recognize a similar need for understanding the other resource management processes. For example, how are supplies, materials, equipment, and tools managed? Is there effective management of the facilities? Are community relations with management appropriate to creating a climate that enables the health care facility to progress?

Financial management, which is usually well understood and accepted as a board responsibility, is in reality only a response to the primary resources--personnel, materials, facilities, and community relations. Because the major expense in the operation of a health care facility is labor, human resources should be the first concern in resource management.

PART II

MANAGEMENT AND THE UNION

INTRODUCTION

MANAGEMENT AND THE UNION

The preceding chapters have presented an overall view of the employee-management relationship and management's responsibilities. Sound employee relations are imperative to the successful administration of any health care facility. A well-managed facility minimizes the possibility of unionization; however, there is always the possibility of a union trying to sell its services or being invited to the institution by several employees. The effective management of labor relations requires knowledge of where and how labor problems arise, as well as of the rights and responsibilities of employees, employers, and the union.

Part II reviews the relationship between management and the union. This section also covers: the election process, bargaining units, how unions can be decertified, post-election management considerations, the collective bargaining process, how to prepare to negotiate a contract, and planning for work stoppages.

It also includes the biggest ethical question of all: the moral obligation of health care employees to care for their patients versus their need to further their own interests via work stoppages.

Additionally, there is a section on the influence of religion on union-management relationship, and some remarks about the positive value of unions.

CHAPTER 7

The Union:
Friend or Foe to Management?

The independent labor union in America dates back before the Civil War, but the labor movement assumed considerable stability with the formation of the American Federation of Labor (AFL) in 1886. In 1935, the present Congress of Industrial Organization (CIO) began its phenomenal growth. The AFL is organized primarily along the lines of crafts, although it does include some industrial unions. The CIO is primarily organized along the lines of general industrial unions. There are many other independent unions not directly affiliated with any particular industry or craft, but the two named are the largest and most powerful.

As a rule, unions prefer to sign trade agreements with employers for an entire industry for either a community, a state, or an entire geographical area. Union growth and strength have changed with the historic tides of prosperity and depression. Although growth of the labor movement in this country from 1786-- through single-plant unions to the Knights of Labor (forerunner of the AFL) and finally to the merger that created the AFL-CIO in 1955--has been accomplished with emotional and some social upheaval, there has been no real deterrence to growth. Unions have been and will continue to be viable enterprises with millions of highly organized and disciplined members, led by trained, educated, and often brilliant men and women.

Although collective bargaining on behalf of health care workers dates back to the 1930s in San Francisco and the 1940s in Minnesota and other areas, union organization tended to lag in the health care field until 1974. From the 1930s to middle 1970s, collective bargaining was a rare happening for health care workers, particularly for health care professionals. Today it is recognized as a means for them to be heard and have their concerns resolved.

The compelling force that drove hospital physicians and private practitioners toward collective bargaining was the perceived intrusion of government and private insurers into the traditional doctor-patient relationship. The driving force for the nurses was wages, staffing patterns, and their demand for professional recognition. For service workers, technicians, and the many others who sought protection through collective bargaining, the issues were pay, working conditions, job security, and fair treatment as individuals.

Major unions currently involved in the health care field are:

- National Union of Hospital and Health Care Employees, District 1199

- Service Employees International Union (SEIU)

- American Federation of State, County, and Municipal Employees (AFSCME)

- American Nurses Association (ANA) & various state nurse associations

- Teamsters

- United Food and Commercial Workers Union

- American Federation of Teachers (AFT).

Unions, like any enterprise, cost money; and they are profit-oriented. The prime source of their money is union members who typically must pay initiation fees to join and regular dues to maintain membership. While the parent union frequently receives a portion of the new member's initiation fee (50 percent is common), its primary source of revenue is the per-capita tax. This is a regular per-member payment made by local unions to the parent union out of the dues they receive from the rank-and-file members. It is estimated that one million unionized health care workers will generate $50 million to $60 million annually in union dues. As a potential source of income, this is certainly an incentive for various unions to want "a piece of the action."

Total revenue received by national and international unions from per-capita dues depends, of course, on two variables, the first being the number of local members, and the second their ability to routinely and consistently pay their dues to the local union.

Without question, unions have exerted a major influence on American industrial complexes in such areas as:

- Wages and benefits, including the establishment of pension plans

- Proper rest room facilities

- Removal of dangerous machinery and/or proper safety guards

- Lunch and rest periods

- Realistic production standards

- Child labor restrictions

- Progressive labor legislation at state and federal levels

- Work simplification methods

- Training and job upgrading.

Although union benefits are intended solely for their members, thousands of nonunion members are today enjoying the fruits of the labor movement. Most union agreements with employers have resulted in increased wages, reduced hours, guaranteed seniority rights, provisions for pension benefits, and provisions for career mobility opportunities not only for unionized facilities but also for many nonunion institutions.

Unionists boast that disputes over organization or contract renewals have been held to a minimum, thus enabling management to concentrate its efforts on higher productivity and efficiency of operation. They also say the cooperative efforts of labor organizations have been instrumental in developing and promulgating the industrial growth of the country.

Opponents to unionism contend that union membership costs employees money and that strike losses are never recouped. Also, they say, members find they have little voice in whether a strike is called or not, and there is little opportunity to find out what the issues really are. Opponents also claim that the employees' fate is regulated by the union hierarchy, and that employees are used to satisfy the economic demands of union leaders.

Many opponents also contend that the most serious adverse effect on employees and the employer's welfare stems from the unions' consistent opposition to the improvement of productivity, on which the lasting success of the business depends. Unions, they say, resist the establishment of incentives to induce employees to work at high levels of efficiency. This "featherbed rule," they claim, results in unneeded employees and payroll expenses for unnecessary or duplicated jobs.

Opponents also argue that instead of encouraging industrial peace and fostering industrial efficiency, active union membership campaigns actually encourage strife and inhibit management's right to strive for greater efficiency in production. They say this in turn inhibits management's ability to make a product and/or deliver a service at a lower cost.

Finally, those opposed to unions contend that, as Keith Davis puts it, "unions show little concern about the side effects of more money, such as inflation, tax increases (when government employees receive more), unfavorable trade balances internationally, and dislocations in the national wage structure."[1]

The basic economic goal of any business is to make a profit. This process includes three basic functions: (1) ownership, (2) management, and (3) the manual effort to produce a product or service. Theoretically, management should act as a go-between for transmitting the policies, projects, and purposes of the entity (ownership) to the workers, and for communicating the capacities and interests of the workers to the governing body. It should perform these functions in such a manner that all the workers, as well as the managers and the institution itself, find their best opportunities fulfilled.

However, the lines of communication between the workers and the entity frequently are complicated and obstructed. This breakdown creates a need that unions are prepared to fill for the workers. The employment relationship becomes more of a business relationship, with a "third party" acting in behalf of a client for a "fee." Therefore, the business of unionism is very much like the business of business.

Few can dispute the fact that in the early years of the labor movement, unionism did contribute significantly to the industrial milieu by improving the economy and working conditions for the American workers. Through the years, as large corporations themselves found ways to "play the game," so have unions found ways to increase the business of unionism for the benefit of interested groups--and their reported efficiency abuses cannot be totally disputed. Unionism does, at times, fuel corporate inefficiency; so, however, do corporations by passiveness that contributes to a need for unionism.

The strongest institutional goals, both for unions and for business, relate to survival. It is when these goals become the ends rather than the means of serving effectively and honestly that one needs to question seriously who is the enemy of management within the labor arena.

UNIONS IN THE HEALTH CARE FIELD:
THE DOWN SIDE

What about the impact of unions in the health care field? What are some of the reasons health care management is opposed to unionization? From the point of view of meeting the responsibility of an effective operation of a health care facility in today's society, there are sound reasons for management to attempt to maintain a direct relationship with employees. The following list, therefore, covers the negative effects of unionization on the management process.

The Negative Effects of Unionization on the Health Care Industry

- Wage increases and fringe-benefit extension and expansion create higher costs. The employee will want some tangible profit from the collective bargaining process after the union dues are withheld.

- Time is lost by the management staff as it copes with union-related problems, contract negotiations, employee orientation to the contract terms, enforcement of the contract, handling of grievances, and preparation for arbitration.

- As management attempts to build a team effort, the union creates a confrontation system, making the employee and management opponents pursuing individual goals rather than teammates with common objectives.

- The cost of union support comes ultimately from the patients or their sources of payments for services rendered. Neither the employee, the patient, nor the institution benefits from the fees, fines, dues, and assessments withheld from employee wages paid to the union. Conversion of time lost to costs creates another indirect cost of union support.

- Health care management lacks the maturity and sophistication to cope in the labor relations field, whereas the union organizers, negotiators, and business agents are often career persons skilled in labor relations practices.

- Involvement of the institution with organized labor in turn involves the facility in all of the National Labor Relations Board decisions, which constitute an entire new body of common-law practice that has its own special impact on future relations with employees.

- The union must have access to the facility to police their contract. This is a form of control over the institution, with no reverse means by which the facility has any control over the union.

- In contract negotiations, it often becomes necessary to satisfy the union and the union representative rather than to satisfy the employees of the institution. Employees may gain or lose, depending upon the union strategy for their overall programs.

- Since collective bargaining does not require that the employer agree to every demand, there is always the danger, despite the special provisions of the NLRA as amended, for strikes, pickets, demonstrations, intimidation, threats, work slowdowns, work stoppages, and other forms of work disruption.

- The union often becomes the objective rather than the means toward better employee relations. The process of negotiation is based on a balanced power, and there is often the need to gain further power to assure satisfactory negotiations.

- Management's basic rights gradually erode with each new negotiated contract. Changes in policies, procedures, methods, and equipment become subject to advance union approval, union review, and possible modification of contract terms as a result of such changes. The union does not take management's rights, but through collective action nullifies management's opportunity to use them, so that the union becomes a party to or a voice in the exercise of such rights without assuming responsibility. Some of the rights affected are the rights to:

- Hire employees without being subject to union referral, union approval, or required union membership.

- Discharge or fire employees for cause without being subject to union review, union appeal, and possible arbitration.

- Promote or transfer employees based on demonstrable merit rather than as a result of forced recognition of seniority.

- Establish the job, determine what should be done, how, when, why, and by whom, without confronting job jurisdictional problems, challenges to procedural changes, modifications of technological method, etc.

- Set the performance standards to determine the quality, quantity, cost, and other conditions for performance without becoming subject to quotas and other conditions.

- Evaluate performance based on the performance standards and take corrective action or discipline without becoming subject to union review, union appeal, and possible arbitration.

- Set wages and determine benefits and personnel policies. The law guarantees the union the right to negotiate wages, hours, and working conditions.

- Initiate changes in policies, procedures, methods, equipment, etc., without becoming subject to advanced union approval, union review, and possible modification of contract terms as a result of such change.

- Freely schedule hours, shifts, and tours of duties without being subject to premium pay and penalty conditions.

- Assign or deploy workers without limitation for job jurisdiction or premium pay.

- Receive, review, and process grievances directly with the employees rather than through a shop steward or committee.

- Reward meritorious performance as an incentive or recognition of an employee without establishing conditions that become negotiable in the next bargaining agreement.

These are but some of the implications of a union on management that suggest that maintaining a nonunion status can promote the efficient and effective operation of the institution. There are many other impacts that could likewise be cited.

Unions in and of themselves do not hinder or enhance productivity. Management has a responsibility to make an effort to enlist unions as partners in enhancing productivity. Unions today are sophisticated enough and intelligent enough to know that a health care facility that goes bankrupt will not benefit them or their members. On the other hand, if management excludes a union from the productivity process, the union still has the strike weapon to use if it doesn't agree with the unilateral program that management wants to implement. Neither strike nor bankruptcy is acceptable. Communication and partnership seem a small price to pay for enhancing productivity. Unions can be a partner to productivity.

POSITIVE VALUE OF UNIONS FOR EMPLOYEES

"Union," in years past, was a dirty word. But in the health care field, unionism of health care workers is no longer the controversial subject it was ten years ago.

American trade unionism has always sought higher wages, better benefits, and shorter hours. Because these are usually popular public issues, they receive the most attention from the news media. As a result, the general public perceives that unions pursue rather narrow economic objectives. Today, that is not entirely true. Labor is showing a lot of maturity in its sense of responsibility to both the organization and the community.

In addition to support on wage and benefit issues for their members, unions have been instrumental in providing working men and women with job security and dignity. They have also curbed discrimination and promoted social legislation aimed at bettering the American way of life. In addition, unions have helped improve working conditions and the quality of supervision within the work environment. In the words of two commentators, "It is easy for health care administrators and supervisors to label the unions as troublemakers, agitators, outside power-mongers, and liars, but another thing for supervisors to see their own faults as reasons for the current success by labor unions to organize health care employees."[2]

MANAGEMENT, THE UNION, RELIGION, AND THE WORKER

Some religious leaders see labor organization and collective bargaining as moral issues, while others see them solely as matters of economic and social concern. In reality they are both, for when management is challenged in its opposition to unionization, what began as an economic and social issue takes on overtones of conscience and morality. What, then, is the relationship among management, religion, unions, and workers?

All are generally concerned with the well-being of the workers. Workers have not only specified moral and legal rights, but also human dignity that both management and unions must respect. The individual worker should not be victimized by the actions or lack of actions of management any more than through the activities of the union, whether in the organizing campaign efforts, during the collective bargaining and negotiating processes, or in the period of working under a labor agreement.

Rights of Management, the Union, and the Worker

It is logical for churches to maintain an interest in protecting the worker from a violation of moral rights. The National Labor Relations Act and the National Labor Relations Board are the means of protecting the employee from the violation of legal rights. The law identifies what those rights are and establishes provisions for unfair labor charges when they are violated. Perhaps one of the most important functions of a union seeking the organization of the workforce of a given employer is to make known to that workforce the rights as they exist and by appropriate monitoring of management's behavior call to the attention of the workers any violation of those rights caused by management. The worker has a right to protect himself and can file his own complaint with the NLRB. On the other hand, the union representative, as a specialist in labor relations and as a self-appointed representative of the employee during the organizing effort, can also file an unfair labor charge against management.

Management finds itself in relatively the same posture of needing to know what the union does so as to protect employees from unfair practices by the union. Management also has the right to file unfair labor charges on behalf of its workforce.

Neither management nor the union, however, has the right to intimidate, to coerce or to threaten the employee. The employee has the stated right to seek representation, join a union, file a petition for an election and to vote in the free and open election as an exercise of conscience. That same worker has the implied right to represent himself, to remain outside of the union, and in the event that there is an NLRB sponsored election, to vote in opposition to the union.

Both management and the union have the right to inform the employee, to present basic issues, to point out the deficiencies of the other party, to examine the track record, and to try to persuade the employee. Neither management nor the union will know the effectiveness of its information and attempts at persuasion until the NLRB has closed the election, counted the votes, and made the results known to all parties concerned.

Role of Religion

From a moral point of view, it would seem that religion must also be concerned for the protection of the workers' moral rights. During the process of information and persuasion, the worker has a right to his personal human dignity, a right to his privacy of person, a right to assemble with others, and a right to exercise his own conscience.

But unlike the NLRB, religion has no established mechanism by which to confront the parties in order to hear their positions, the actions pursued, and the results intended. There is no mechanism by which both sides can confront each other in the presence of religious leadership and await judgment. There is the tendency for some religious leaders, serving often as self-appointed spokesmen, to express a personal viewpoint as the position of the church and to relate that point of view through either known information or allegation that might be made about the other party. It is perhaps unfortunate that management seldom asks any religious leaders for advice or support. Union leadership, on the other hand, often asks for and expects religious leaders to exercise some unique support for the union's position. It is therefore highly selective as to which spokesmen within a particular religious party it wants to have on its side, seeking spokesmen who support the position they have taken and not running the risk of choosing an opponent.

THE CHOICES

Several sound arguments support management's right to oppose the unionization of its workforce, provided it does not interfere with the employees' inherent moral and legal rights.

- **Protecting the public.** Unions, from their inception as trade guilds, have been an economic and social phenomena. In the beginning they were benevolent, providing for the protection of their membership. Their basic aim through collective bargaining was the just distribution of the profits after both management and the employee had received a fair share for their risk and their input. As the unions grew in numbers and in strength, they became more than a voluntary banding together of a group of employees to protect themselves under one employer. They developed political overtones by attempting to do through law what they could not do at the bargaining table.

This political significance continues today, and the bargaining process covers more than the distribution of profits. Today the result of collective bargaining is the determination of the amount of increased costs for services or products produced and the price structure. It is no longer management that pays more than it intended, but the public that ultimately must pay more as a result of the collective bargaining agreement. There are moral implications not only of the wages to be paid, but also of the prices that must be charged in order to pay negotiated wages. Protection of the public from unjust prices has as much moral implication as the protection of the workforce from unjust wages.

- **Alternatives.** With or without unions, there are controls against monopolies in business, but there are no controls against monopolies in unions. Employers, if they are to survive in a free market, can deviate only so far from the mainstream of competition in wages, benefits and working conditions or find that they can neither retain employees nor recruit replacements of the same quality and capacity. Inferior wages, benefits, and working conditions tend to attract inferior performers; inferior performers bring into business or a health care institution a host of other problems: low morale, high absenteeism, excessive labor turnover, inadequate response to training, poor safety practices, and frequent complaints. In a sense, the coexistence of the union versus nonunion workforce establishes a baseline for both management and workers to judge the appropriateness of the wages, benefits, and working conditions established by a given employer. There must be some approximation of fairness.

  A union is no means of achieving a just relationship between the worker and management. There are alternatives, however. Enlightened management is as sound a means as a union. Government itself has become another alternate means to established agencies for the protection of the worker, even subjecting the employer to review, inspection, and litigation where fault is alleged and supported by initial evidence. Although one means might be preferable to another in a particular situation, all three of these options could have the desired result.

- **Inhibiting "community."** The concept of "community" recognizes the interdependence and interrelationship of all. A true community is based on mutuality of need and commonality of purpose. There must be no significance in either dependency or independency, but rather a striving toward an appropriate system of mutual support through recognized interdependence.

Translating the sense of community to the workplace, management needs the workforce and the workforce equally needs good management. There is a commonality of purpose and a mutual respect of needs. As the worker must satisfactorily meet management's requirements, so must the worker be satisfied by management's response to basic needs. The end product is both a satisfactory and a satisfied employee.

By unionizing a given group of employees, organized labor actually inhibits that sense of community that society wants and management must have to be fully successful. The union in practice becomes a force of opposition challenging the positions of management, verbalizing complaints about management's actions or lack of actions, and then confronting management through the collective bargaining process and eventually through the grievance system, including arbitration. What occurs then is a system of organized opposition and confrontation that often leads to conflict through work stoppages and strikes.

What is needed is a system of cooperation leading to collaboration. Although some unions profess that this is their goal, there are few examples to illustrate that it is achievable under the direction of the large national and international unions that seem to have grown apart from the needs and desires of their own memberships.

- **Loss of trust.** Because of the need to separate the idealism from the reality of unionization and collective bargaining, the presence of a union tends to set aside or submerge such virtues as openness, honesty, trust and freedom, rather than enhance them. There is difficulty in maintaining a spirit of openness, since whatever is said or done by either side is subject to challenge, repudiation, or even unfair labor charges. Honesty is often questioned, particularly in the way union pamphlets and management handouts rebut each other. The longer the campaign to persuade the employees, the greater the likelihood employees will mistrust both management and union. The trust needed to maintain a healthy relationship is sometimes the victim of the unionizing effort. The sense of freedom is lost during the union campaign, as limitations are placed on both management and union. In the end, whoever wins, there are often two camps not merely between the workforce and management, but also among the employees themselves. "Winners versus losers" is not the way to establish a true sense of teamwork, oneness, or community.

- **Factors beyond negotiation.** Finally, many of the issues that prompt employee interest in a union become nonnegotiable factors. By law the union can negotiate wages (both cash and benefit), hours, and working conditions, but the real problem is the absence of or breakdown in communication and basic human relationships. In labor-management relations the predominant forces that stimulate interest in unionization are insecurity, a lack of confidence in management, and strained relationships. The factors most conducive to a nonunion situation, then, would seem to be a realistic sense of security, confidence in management's leadership, and harmonious relationships.

Security can be partially economic, but it might also be social, psychological, physical, moral, and managerial. Although the union can negotiate higher wages, greater benefits, and certain restrictions on management behavior, there is little that can be negotiated that will deal with moral, psychological, and physical insecurities. If the workers do not like their manager before a union election, there is no reason to assume at the bargaining table that they will learn to like that manager. There is no way to negotiate openness, honesty, trust, freedom, or mutual respect. There can be no contractual guarantee of full and open communication, nor can the collective bargaining process ensure harmonious and satisfactory relationships among employees or between the workforce and the supervisors and higher levels of management. These conditions tend to result from cooperative human effort, not from the negotiating process.

A POSITIVE APPROACH

The best opposition to the collective bargaining process is not in fighting the workers but in fighting the causes of poor relationships, loss of competence, and creation of insecurities. Positive personnel practices are essential for enlightened management. Careful recruitment, screening, selection and placement of the worker in the right job are all necessary. Enhancing the ability to perform by adequate orientation, appropriate job instruction, training, and programs aimed at continued education and personal development are essential. Adequate counseling, continuous communication, and appropriate employee participation in decision making are all elements of a sound program of enlightened management.

Management has already established its track record. Constant review and auditing of that record is important. If the worker can become disenchanted with management's track record, the union can identify the deficiencies and use as its primary weapon management's own performance. When management has corrected its deficiencies and created a true sense of teamwork, it has little cause for concern about the unionization or nonunion status of its work force.

Regardless of what management has or has not done, there will be some employees who by cultural conviction feel they need and want a union. There will be others with a sufficient sense of insecurity to desire a source of protection. Conversely, there will be those who believe that collective bargaining is not worthy of their human dignity and that they can provide their own vehicle for attaining a voice in their work destiny. Regardless, however, of the beliefs or causes, when there is an active effort to persuade employees to join a union, seek union representation, file a petition, and vote affirmatively in an NLRB election, there must be equal opportunity for management to pursue a process of persuasion. Appropriate information to employees is crucial, so that when an individual employee presents himself to the NLRB deputy and is issued an official ballot to vote, that vote will be a matter of an informed conscience and not the result of having been victimized by one side or the other or emotionalized by intimidation.

THE ETHICAL QUESTION

The most pressing ethical question among health care workers who become involved in labor disputes relates to their moral obligation to care for their patients versus their need to further their own interest through strikes or work stoppages. Since the passage of the Taft-Hartley Amendments in August 1974, there have been numerous strikes by health care workers. They have withheld their services for more money, better hours, more benefits, patient care issues, and health safety concerns. Even physicians have gone on strike to protest their working conditions.

The ethical question, although considered each time there is a labor dispute, is resolved much more quickly today than several years ago. Harry Schwartz expressed it this way:

"I shall not take the absolutist attitude that all strikes in the health care industry are illegal and immoral and should be prohibited, nor shall I take the differentiated position that only certain strikes by certain categories of health care workers are justified while others are completely unjustified. I think a rational patient or potential patient must recognize that we have entered a new era in health industry labor relations, and that no amount of handwringing, repeating of old saws and moralisms, or other inappropriate exhibitionism is going to change the situation."[3]

ENDNOTES

1. Keith Davis, Ph.D., *Human Relations at Work*, Third Edition. New York: McGraw Hill, 1967, page 240.

2. Warren H. Chaney and Thomas R. Beech, *The Union Epidemic*. Rockville, MD: Aspen Publications, 1976.

3.   Harry Schwartz, Ph.D. State University of New York, Appendix A--Taft-Hartley Amendments--Implications for the Health Care Field, Public Viewpoint Seminar, Chicago: American Hospital Association, 1976.

CHAPTER 8

Basic Components of the Union Election Process: Bargaining Units and Decertification

Once a labor organization has begun its organization attempt, the organizer has employees sign authorization cards (See Exhibit 8-1), which in effect often serve as union membership applications as well as authorization of the union to act as the exclusive agent for the employee. Once the union convinces 30 percent of the employees in an appropriate bargaining unit[1] to sign authorization cards, it may send a representation petition to the appropriate regional branch of the NLRB. Prior to receiving a copy of the representation petition, the facility may also receive a recognition demand letter, in which the union states that it represents the majority of the employees in an appropriate bargaining unit. Management usually declines to recognize the union on the basis of the recognition demand letter alone and will refer it to the National Labor Relations Board to file a petition.

Once the petition is filed, the facility has several weeks to decide whether it will sign an election consent agreement or demand a hearing on appropriate unit or other issues. If the facility consents, the election is usually held about a month after the signing of the consent agreement. If a hearing is held, the NLRB's regional director will usually decide the issues within several months. If he decides an election is required, the election date is set for about a month after his decision.

After the election date is set, the facility is required to submit an Excelsior List,[2] which is a list of the names and addresses of all the employees in the bargaining unit. The election itself is usually held on the premises and is conducted by secret ballot (See Exhibit 8-2). During the balloting, there are present one or more observers from each side plus an agent of the National Labor Relations Board. The results of the election are based solely on the majority of the votes cast, not the numbers of employees in the unit.

BASICS OF SOLICITATION AND DISTRIBUTION

In the realm of solicitation/distribution, employees have certain rights during the organizing process (See Exhibit 8-3).

UNION AUTHORIZATION CARD

BUSINESS REPLY MAIL

First Class Permit No. 634   New Haven, Connecticut

COMMUNICATIONS WORKERS OF AMERICA - AFL-CIO

2911 DIXWELL AVENUE

HAMDEN, CONNECTICUT 06518

 1

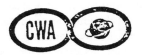 COMMUNICATIONS WORKERS
OF AMERICA, AFL-CIO

(PRINT) Last Name	First		Middle
Street & Number	City	State	Zip
Tel. No.	Job Title & Work Location		Shift

I am an Employee of _____
and I hereby designate the Communications Workers of America, as my
collective bargaining representative.

Date	Signature

Representation Authorization

Exhibit 8-1.

```
+---------------------------------------------------------------+
|                   UNITED STATES OF AMERICA                    |
|                 National Labor Relations Board                |
|                                                               |
|             OFFICIAL SECRET BALLOT                            |
|                   For certain employees of                    |
+---------------------------------------------------------------+
| Do you wish to be represented for purposes of collective      |
| bargaining by -                                               |
|                                                               |
|                        SAMPLE                                 |
|                                                               |
+---------------------------------------------------------------+
|            MARK AN "X" IN THE SQUARE OF YOUR CHOICE            |
|                                                               |
|            YES                          NO                    |
|            [ ]                          [ ]                   |
+---------------------------------------------------------------+
```

DO NOT SIGN THIS BALLOT Fold and drop in ballot box.
If you spoil this ballot return it to the Board Agent for a new one.

FORM NLRB-707N2 (RC, RM, RD CASES) (3-81)

Exhibit 8-2.

Definitions

Solicitation: The practice, act, or instance of approaching an employee and expressing union views to that employee or asking him/her to take a certain action or to sign an authorization card. An employee can be solicited orally, in writing or by a combination of both.

Distribution: The wholesale handing out of leaflets and handbills.

Outsiders: Those individuals who are not employees of the facility.

Employees: Those individuals employed by the facility.

Work time: Includes the working time of both the employee doing the soliciting and distributing and the employee to whom it is directed. Lunch time and rest periods are not ''working time'' no matter how short

Form NLRB–4722
(10–70)

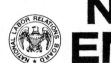

NOTICE TO EMPLOYEES

POSTED PURSUANT TO A SETTLEMENT AGREEMENT APPROVED BY A REGIONAL DIRECTOR OF THE NATIONAL LABOR RELATIONS BOARD
AN AGENCY OF THE UNITED STATES GOVERNMENT

The National Labor Relations Act gives all employees these rights:

> To engage in self-organization;
> To form, join, or assist unions;
> To bargain collectively through repre-
> sentatives of their own choosing;
> To act together for collective bargain-
> ing or other mutual aid or protection;
> To refrain from any and all of these
> activities.

WE WILL NOT restrain or coerce our employees in the exercise of the aforementioned rights. More specifically,

WE WILL NOT promulgate, maintain or enforce any rule or regulation which prohibits our employees from soliciting on behalf of any labor organization on hospital premises, other than immediate patient care areas, during employees' non-working time, or from distributing literature on behalf of any labor organization in non-work areas of our hospital during their non-working time, unless special circumstances and needs of the hospital require such restrictions. Our employees are free to engage in such solicitation and dis-tribution in the coffee shop, cafeteria and employee and public parking lots of the hospital.

WE WILL NOT in any like or related manner interfere with, restrain or coerce employees in the exercise of the right to engage in Union or concerted activities for the purpose of mutual aid or protection as guaranteed in Section 7 of the Act, or to refrain from any and all such activities.

WE WILL expunge from our employee handbook or posted notices anything contrary to this notice.

_____
(Employer)

DATED:

THIS IS AN OFFICIAL NOTICE AND MUST NOT BE DEFACED BY ANYONE

This notice must remain posted for 60 consecutive days from the date of posting and must not be altered, defaced, or covered by any other material. Any questions concerning this notice or compliance with its provisions may be directed to the Board's Office.

Exhibit 8-3.

or irregularly scheduled and regardless of whether the employee is paid for the time.

Work areas: Those areas not defined as nonwork areas.

Nonwork Areas: Could include employee lounges, rest rooms, parking lots, stairways, cafeteria, canteen, and sidewalks.

Patient care areas: Patient rooms, patient treatment rooms, and other areas where solicitation may pose a substantial threat to patient tranquility.

General Rules Related to Solicitation and Distribution

In order to minimize disruption to the operation of the facility, interference with patient care, and inconvenience to the patients and visitors, the following rules will usually apply to solicitation and distribution of literature:

Outsiders: Absent special circumstances, may not solicit for any purpose or distribute any literature on the facility's property at any time. Outsiders are free to hand out literature and solicit workers on public property.

Employees: May not *solicit* for any purpose during working time or in *patient care areas.* Employees may not *distribute literature* for any purpose during *working time* or in patient care or *working areas.*

Bulletin Boards

If a health care facility allows nonemployee groups such as civic, political or commercial groups to post material on its bulletin boards, it may be required to allow a union to use the boards in a like manner. Likewise, if an employer allows employees to post notices of interest to them, without some control parameters, the employer cannot lawfully forbid the same employees to post union notices.

Discriminatory Enforcement

Discriminatory enforcement of a presumptively valid no solicitation/no distribution rule can be unlawful. An employer may not ban *union* organizers and officials from its premises while permitting substantial solicitation and distribution by other nonemployees. It should enforce the rule against all nonemployees in a uniform, nondiscriminatory manner. Similarly, a rule banning employee solicitation and distribution should apply to *all* employee solicitation and not just union activities.

Union Buttons and Insignias

Generally, employees have the right to wear union buttons or other insignia demonstrating their support for unions. However, in special circumstances relating to issues such as safety and the impact on patients and/or visitors, nondiscriminatory restrictions may be upheld.

BARGAINING UNITS

There has been a great deal of litigation concerning appropriate bargaining units for employees in health care institutions. There are no statutory provisions specifically applicable to health care bargaining units. The controversy has centered on concern expressed during the congressional reports and hearings that led to the passage of the 1974 health care amendments that unit fragmentation in health care institutions would increase labor disputes and disrupt or adversely affect patient care.[3] The legislative history most frequently quoted concerning this issue is the statement contained in Senate and House committee reports that "[d]ue consideration should be given by the Board to preventing proliferation of bargaining units in the health care industry."[4] The Congressional debates that preceded passage of the 1974 amendments supported the directive against proliferation of bargaining units in health care institutions.

In December 1982 the NLRB issued a lengthy explanation of its initial approach to analysis of health care bargaining units. IN *St. Francis Hospital*,[5] 265 NLRB No. 120, 112 LRRM 1153, the NLRB delineated a two-tiered procedure for determining the appropriateness of health care bargaining units. As a first step, the NLRB usually determined whether the requested unit fell into one of the seven enumerated categories identified as commonly found in health care institutions: (1) physicians, (2) registered nurses, (3) other professional employees, (4) technical employees, (5) business office clerical employees, (6) service and maintenance employees, and (7) skilled maintenance employees. Upon determining that the unit fit one of these classifications, the NLRB applied traditional unit principles to determine whether the specific employees involved displayed the requisite community of interest to warrant separate representation. If a union sought to represent a unit of employees smaller than one of the seven identified groups, the NLRB usually dismissed the petition before it went into the second stage of analysis unless presented with extraordinary and compelling facts justifying allowance of a smaller unit.

After several Circuit Courts criticized these unit determination principles on the ground that they did not sufficiently take into account congressional concern over undue unit proliferation, the NLRB reversed itself and in 1984 promulgated a new approach in a case called *St. Francis II*, 271 NLRB No. 160, 116 LRRM 1465. This new approach stipulated that in order to have any unit smaller than either all professional order to have any unit smaller than either all professional or all nonprofessional employees, there must exist sharper than usual disparities between the terms and conditions of employment of those employees sought by the union and the remainder of the employees. While the new *St. Francis II* approach will doubtless result in fewer and larger units, the exact meaning of "sharper than usual disparities" has not yet been articulated by the NLRB.5

More unit determination litigation can be expected as more health care employees find themselves out of the traditional acute care hospital setting and into new work environments such as home care services, health maintenance organizations, congregate housing programs, skilled nursing facilities, emergi-centers and so on. Among other things the labor complements in these new health care delivery systems are small, and the NLRB in deciding appropriateness of unit will therefore most likely need to take into account relevant differences from large hospitals.

The determination of the appropriate unit is the most important aspect of a union organizing effort. It can generally be assumed that the union has already computed the number of employees and attempted to devise a voting group in which it feels it has a substantial opportunity to win an election. This presents opportunities for an employer to attempt to change the voting group in hopes of weakening the union. The issues that may be raised in the course of unit determination are so varied that it is difficult to summarize them all. However, some of the issues that can be raised are:

- expanding the voting group to include other facilities of the same health care facility

- supervisory challenges, as Section 2(11) of the NLRA defines supervisors as part of management (See Exhibit 8-4)

- expanding the unit to include part-time employees

- increasing the size of the unit to include all employees at a particular facility if the union is seeking only a limited group.

Many factors can go into establishing an appropriate unit. The most significant consideration with respect to all these factors is that they are substantially in the control of the employer. This fact, which has been criticized by some of the more union-oriented, creates substantial opportunities for an employer to organize its operation to decrease the possibility of successful union organizing.

DETERMINING SUPERVISORY STATUS
WITHIN THE MEANING OF SEC. 2(11)
OF THE NATIONAL LABOR RELATIONS ACT

Test #1

The NLRB has generally recognized the following primary tests in determining supervisory status. It must be emphasized, however, that all listed criteria need *not* be met in order to be treated as a supervisor. A supervisor may:

Hire	Transfer
Suspend	Lay off
Recall	Promote
Discharge	Assign work
Reward	Discipline
Direct	Adjust grievances

Test #2

The definition of ''supervisor'' in the NLRA lists some important functions that set the supervisor apart from other employees. In many borderline cases, however, the NLRB and the courts have looked to various secondary test of supervisory status. Among facts that have been regarded as weighing in favor of supervisory status are the following:

- Designation as a charge person or supervisor,
- is regarded by himself or others as a supervisor,
- has privileges accorded only to supervisors,
- attends instructional sessions or meetings held for supervisory personnel,
- is responsible for a shift or phase of operations, (clinic, health entity),
- receives orders from management rather than from other supervisors,
- has authority to interpret or transmit employer's instructions to other employees,
- has responsibility for inspecting the work of others,
- gives instructions to other employees,
- has authority to grant or deny leave of absence,
- has responsibility for reporting policy infractions,
- keeps time records on other employees,
- records of time worked is differently from other employees,
- authorizes overtime work,
- is paid differently from other employees.

Exhibit 8-4.

This kind of opportunity often arises in the case of an employer that operates more than one facility. In such circumstances, it is sometimes possible to structure an employer's operation so that a single facility would be determined to be inappropriate for purposes of collective bargaining, thereby preventing an election limited to that facility. This is significant because the burden of organizing a group of facilities is much more substantial from the union's point of view, particularly as the fuel for union interest often arises from concerns restricted to employees at a particular facility.

DECERTIFICATION PROCESS

The decertification process is basically the reverse of the election process. Any employee or group of employees on behalf of 30 percent or more of the employees in a unit covered by a collective bargaining contract may at an appropriate time file a petition with the NLRB to rescind the union's authority. The petition must be signed and sworn to, or must contain a declaration by the signer that the contents are true and correct. If the petitioner has shown that the petition is supported by a 30 percent showing of interest,[6] the NLRB will conduct a secret ballot election of employees in the unit. Like a representation election, the results of the election are based solely on the majority of the votes cast, not the numbers of employees in the unit.

An employee decertification petition may not be filed by an employer, nor may the employer sponsor or assist employees in the preparation of such a petition.[7] Such conduct will invalidate the petition. However, in special circumstances an employer may file its own employer representation petition in an attempt to decertify a union. To do so, an employer must have what the NLRB has called "objective" grounds for doubting the union's majority status. Such "objective" grounds usually involve a petition signed by a majority of employees and given to the employer stating that they no longer wish the union to represent them. Employee turnover and even resignation from the union by a majority of employees are not normally considered to be such "objective" grounds.

PREVENTIVE LABOR RELATIONS

Labor relations between health care workers and providers will become more profound, particularly as cost containment pressures force health care facilities to stress productivity, lower staff complements, close or convert beds, promote organizational restructures, join multi-institutions and enter into new marketing ventures.

Keeping up with the rapid changes in labor and employment laws will be a challenging task for health care management. Current labor practice patterns will need to change in the years ahead as the American health care system continues its metamorphosis. In the final analysis, "the essence of preventive labor relations, i.e., avoiding or averting union activity, lies in establishing and maintaining an aggressive employee relations program designed to build employee morale, loyalty and commitment to the goals of the business. Such a program must be initiated long before any signs of union organizing activity and must be maintained with a single-minded dedication."[8] An aggressive employee relations program requires more management effort and attention than any election process.

ENDNOTES

1.   Refers to criteria for including or excluding employees from a voting unit. The National Labor Relations Board considers whether employees have community or similarity of interest and therefore whether they should be included in the same unit (e.g., same job duties and compensation, same overall work flow and overall supervision, same employee facilities, similarity of skills, etc.)

2.   In 1966, the National Labor Relations Board decided in *Excelsior Underwear, Inc.*, 156 NLRB 1236, 61 LRRM 1217, to require employers to furnish unions with list of employees' names and home addresses. The list is used by the union in its organizing efforts at the institution.

3.   U. S. Congress. Senate. Committee on Labor and Public Welfare. Subcommittee on Labor. 93rd Congress, 2d Sess., 1974. (Legislative History of the Nonprofit Hospitals Under the NLRA (1974).

4.   Rep. No. 766, 93rd Congress, 2d Sess. 5 (1974) reprinted in 1974 U.S. Code Cong. & Ad, News 3946, 3950; H.R. Rep. No. 1051, 93rd Cong., 2d Sess. 7 (1974) reprinted in 1974 U.S. Code Cong. & Ad. News 3950.

5.   The NLRB is considering three cases, *Keokuk Area Hospital, North Arundel Hospital Association,* and *Monadnock Community Hospital,* that raise the issue of when a registered nurse unit can be appropriate under the *St. Frances II* approach. In *Southern Maryland Hospital,* 274 NLRB 212, 118 NRRM 1599 (1985), the Board found disparities that justified a technical employees unit in a large (1,200 nonsupervisory employee) hospital; however, in *St. Luke's Memorial Hospital,* 274 NLRB 202, 118 LRRM 1545 (1985), it found insufficient disparities to justify a licensed practical nurses' unit in a substantially smaller hospital.

6.   NLRB Statements of Procedure 101.18(a), 29 CFR 101.18 9(a) (1971).

7.   LMRA 101.19(c)(1)(A). NLRB Rules and Regulations 102.60(a), 29 CFR 102.60(a) (1971). See also *Star Brush Mfg. Co.,* 100 NLRB 679, 30 LRRM 1335 (1952), holding that confidential employees (e.g., executive secretaries) may not file decertification petitions.

8.   Louis Jackson and Robert Lewis. *Winning NLRB Elections.* (New York: Practising Law Institute) 1972.

CHAPTER 9

Post-Election
Management Considerations

Elections cannot be lost if they are not held. On the other hand, there are no real winners in an election. The dissipation of energy, the expense of counsel, the loss of trust, the creation of disharmony, and the fear of retaliation can be problems to management, employees, and the union. To some extent, also, patients may become innocent victims of either management or the union actions. As a means of placing management in the best possible posture within the operation and in terms of future management-employee relations, whether management or union wins, the following is offered:

IF THE EMPLOYER WINS

- **Avoid gloating.** Because of the emotionalism that accompanies most employee organizing efforts, winning stimulates a sense of relief and joy that may be viewed as gloating. The outcome of most elections separates those who supported management from those who did not, and also identifies a third group: those who did not have a commitment either way and who did not want to become involved. It is the union-committed and noncommitted group combined that poses an ongoing threat to management. Often these two groups constitute a majority that must still be won over by management. It is therefore important that management be seen and heard not only by formal communication, such as letters, but in the informal handshakes and verbal expressions of appreciation for the outcome of the election, the need to unify the operation once again, and the need to demonstrate that the confidence placed in administration and the management process is deserved.

- **Enhance credibility.** It is important not only to maintain the credibility of management but to enhance it, particularly among those employees who had no commitment or had a commitment to the union. Among other measures this requires that management preserve its integrity by maintaining all of the effective patterns of behavior utilized during the campaign that stimulated improved employee security, growth in employee confidence in the integrity of management and more open, positive, and harmonious relationships between management personnel and the working employee. Uppermost is the need to maintain and improve the open lines of two-way communication--the means by which management has communicated to the employees and, equally important, the means by which the employees have found it possible to communicate to management. In time these two processes must be blended to become the process of discussion or dialogue that can lead to decision-making and/or problem solving.

- **Reappraise issues.** With the election over, management is not restricted from either the implied or actual benefits of change. It is vital, therefore, that the key management personnel involved in the union campaign effort quickly reappraise all identified issues in the management-employee relationship and work toward a prompt and satisfactory solution. It is possible to achieve this in a way that provides the employees a greater voice in the operation but at the same time preserves management's rights to manage. The democratization of management is inevitable. Authoritarianism and autocratic behavior must be viewed as obsolete.

- **Reexamine management structure.** To maintain management's right to manage, there is an obligation to manage effectively. It is therefore crucial that the entire management structure and process be reexamined objectively--which may require some hard decisions. Among some key questions that must be raised and answered are:

  - Is there a clear identification of administration (program management, which may include both line and staff programs), departmental and/or functional management, and unit supervision?

  - What lessons have been learned from the union activity that indicate weaknesses of both general and specific types in these three levels of management?

  - To what extent do present job descriptions delineate the necessary management tasks?

  - To what extent is there need for more effective monitoring of board administration or administration over department directors with regard to appropriate performance of management tasks?

  - In what way and to what extent has the management process held subordinates accountable?

  - To what extent are there recognized and established performance standards known by the superior and the subordinate at each level of management to guide both performance and evaluation of performance?

- To what extent do management personnel understand and accept the responsibilities of the management role and process in the organization?

- Is there need for specific training in how to manage or specific education to acquire the competency to manage?

- Is there a sense of harmony and unity within the various levels of management--administration, department management, and supervision?

- Is there a sense of peer support and a commonality of interest?

- To what extent is there a sense of unity or harmony that makes management a team?

- **Study employee programs.** There is need to study very carefully employee-related programs, systems, policies, and procedures and to evaluate net effectiveness in terms of the intended objectives versus the actual results. Included in this examination should be:

  - A review of the means by which wages are determined for particular jobs to verify the internal and external equity of wage rates and to ensure that appropriate pay to individual employees is maintained.

  - An examination of the adequacy of the present package of benefits. Does the competitive posture of local commerce and industry give rise to a negative comparison between what the health care facility provides and what employees expect?

  - An evaluation of the appropriateness of the performance criteria used for the recruitment, screening, and selection process. The work should be under such control that the process can specify the nature of the worker appropriate for performance.

  - A reexamination of both the adequacy and effectiveness of the present programs of employee orientation (introduction to the work and work environment), job training (learning how to apply one's competency to the tasks assigned), and continuing education (the acquisition of additional knowledge, skills, and other competencies for growth, development, and eventual promotion).

  - A review of the present systems of employee counseling and means of follow-up plus documentation. Are both the facility and the employees adequately protected based on records retained? Are personnel files complete? Are forms properly completed, signed, and filed? Are all documents, forms, and other records centralized?

- A reexamination of the performance appraisal system. Are there realistic performance standards against which an objective performance appraisal can be executed? Is the present performance appraisal form appropriate to benefit both the employee and management? Does it lead to a sense of security for the employee, with implied benefit resulting from continued improvement? Is the supervisor adequately appraising performance and counseling employees with regard to such appraisal, and is this process adequately monitored by higher levels of management to assure success? What is the final disposition of performance appraisals?

- Are personnel policies understood and accepted by both management personnel and the employees? Do they establish a positive environment for working relationships? Is there adequate means for review and revision? Are terms defined? Is there protection from too many exceptions? Is there assurance of consistency in interpretation and enforcement? Is there a clear delineation between hospital policy and what is acceptable as departmental policy?

- **Assessments by professionals.** Professional assessments of relative strengths and weaknesses in other aspects of the hospital's operational program might have their own specific value at this point. For example:

  - The assessment of the relative strengths and weaknesses of management practice from the point of view of the employee--an employee attitude or morale survey--is a quick way to ascertain problems that employees see.

  - A professional audit of the personnel administration program, and the way in which it is actually managed by the department managers and supervisors, could have the same value for the continued management of human resources as a financial management audit would have for the continued management of financial resources.

  - An image study might serve as a general assessment of the facility as a source of health care services, health care education, or an employer. The points of view of physicians, past and present patients, civic and business leaders, employees, volunteers, church authorities, and other segments of the public could be a valued tool for future operational planning, for revitalized public relations both internally and externally, and for achievement of a closer alliance of the hospital to the local community by identifying the ways in which each is dependent on the other.

It is hoped that the foregoing points will be helpful in a systematic review of the operations, and that the result will be a more positive and productive operation that protects the health care facility from another confrontation.

IF THE UNION WINS

At the beginning of every NLRB election, both the health care facility and the union anticipate a victory--but only one will win. In the event that the union is the victor, a number of special considerations are suggested to guide management. Keep in mind that management at this point needs to present a posture of conviction and integrity that will support its position during the collective bargaining process. Weakness in any form at this point must be avoided. The following points are offered, therefore, as immediate guides:

- **Reexamine the management team.** The most essential single action is the reexamination and reconstruction of the management team. This requires careful study of who does what, and in what relationship, to effectively manage the operation.

- **Communicate regret.** Communicate both formally and informally to employees management's regret with the outcome of the election and concern over the intervention of a third party in the management-employee relationship. Management can no longer take unilateral action to resolve its problems.

- **Postmortem.** There is need for a serious postmortem to reappraise all that has been learned from the inception of the current union activity to the outcome of the election. It is suggested that there be three separate groups: administration, the concerned departmental managers, and the concerned middle- and first-line supervisors. These groups should explore chronologically the cause and effect of each situation that developed or occurred. What happened or what failed to happen that permitted negative situations to arise or persist? Why was management insensitive or nonperceptive to the reality of these negative conditions? Where, how, why, when, and with whom did the communication process fail? What actions did the employees expect from management that were not forthcoming? What aspects of the union campaign proved to be inappropriate or ineffective?
Once each level of management separately evaluates the entire period of union activity, a joint conference should be planned. This should lead

to the identification of specific operational problems and a plan of action to overcome such problems and thus maximize management's chances at the bargaining table. The outcome of this postmortem should be management's understanding of what was not known that should have been known, what was misinterpreted that misguided management, what actions or decisions were not taken that would have changed the outcome, and what specific management positions must be protected at the bargaining table.

- **Avoid negative actions.** Management must avoid the temptation to pursue any negative actions that might be construed as reprisal, revenge, or retaliation. The employees have formally confronted management and have won. The need to win friends among the union-committed group is still vital.

- **Prepare for collective bargaining.** Prepare management to receive the initial opening demands and to proceed with the collective bargaining process. Determine who will be the chief negotiator and who will serve as additional members of the negotiating team. Identify those management rights that must be preserved intact, those that can be modified, and the extent of modification acceptable. Establish negotiating limits on wages, benefits, hours, and other matters related to working conditions that will require separate administrative and board of trustee review and approval before pursuit at the bargaining table. Identify those conditions vital to effective control of the operation, and maintenance of management's authority commensurate with its responsibility. Establish the means of exercising accountability once the contract is negotiated, ratified, and signed.

- **Watch prenegotiating agreements.** Be cautious of prenegotiation agreements that may set precedents or limit freedom at the bargaining table. The union may demand that the facility pay members of the negotiating team regular wages during the negotiating process. The union may expect the employer to cover the cost of the facilities for negotiation meetings. There may be suggestions for a separate agreement for compulsory arbitration to avoid any strike action during the initial contract negotiation. There may even be a suggested agreement that arbitration will deal only with the last best offer from either side. Any number of issues might serve as content for a prenegotiating agreement. Each has advantages and disadvantages and must therefore be carefully studied in the light of the facility's overall objectives for the collective bargaining process.

An employer who has a union, in essence, has a partner in the business. But union elections always have an aftermath of mistrust, hard feelings, dissension, and fear of retaliation by both sides. The union unites the employees. It does not unite the management-employee relationship. Management should consider the post-election period a time to make a fresh start and begin working toward improvements in labor relations.

CHAPTER 10

The Collective Bargaining Process

PROCEDURES AND ISSUES

If a labor organization is successful in gaining recognition as the exclusive bargaining agent for employees within an appropriate bargaining unit, management is legally required to sit down and bargain "in good faith" with representatives of the union.

Section 8(d) of the National Labor Relations Act sets forth the ground rules for collective bargaining. Essentially, it is the mutual obligation of the employer and the union to meet at "reasonable times" and to confer "in good faith" with respect to wages, hours, and other terms and conditions of employment. Emphasis must be placed on "good faith," as this is an obligation dictated by law and imposed on both parties during negotiations. This does not mean that management must agree with the union or accept any particular union proposal, and "hard bargaining" is lawful. But it does require that management negotiate with the goal of reaching a contract, not thwarting one.

The process of bargaining in the health care field, like bargaining in any other industry, basically consists of the presentation of demands by the union and of counterproposals advanced by management, with the objective of reaching a set of agreeable compromises resulting in a signed final agreement.

The bargaining process usually takes place outside the facility. The institution is normally represented by a "chief spokesperson" (usually a labor attorney or labor relations consultant), by the facility's personnel director, and perhaps by another member of upper management. The union's negotiating committee is usually headed by the local business agent, or frequently by a union attorney. In addition, bargaining unit employees will be at the bargaining table. These employees are usually elected by their fellow workers and tend to be outspoken supporters of the union. Quite frequently, the employees at the bargaining table are those who first initiated union activities within the institution.

Prior to any bargaining, each side will conduct internal strategy sessions to review which issues are to be discussed and which issues can and cannot be compromised. The union generally develops a list of demands. Often the union demands closely parallel the key issues discussed during the union's organizational drive and represent the concerns expressed to the union by dissatisfied workers. The demands commonly include wage increases, improved employee benefits, and job security. Moreover, in health care, far more than in traditional industry, the union's proposals will often call for employee involvement in the decision- and policy-making process.

The law requires that management at least negotiate with the union about issues involving employee wages and working conditions. These are termed "mandatory" subjects of bargaining. To the extent, however, that the union's proposals stray too far from these basic issues and intrude on such normal management prerogatives as the selection of supervisors or general policy-making for the facility, management may be within its rights in refusing even to discuss such topics, which are termed "permissive" subjects of bargaining. In fact, while it is legal for a party to "bargain to impasse" over a mandatory subject, it is illegal to do so over a "permissive subject" (that is, to refuse to conclude a contract because of insistence on a nonmandatory subject).

Management usually receives the demands of the union and the arguments in support of the demands at the first negotiating session. It then prepares to respond and to offer counterproposals at the subsequent negotiating sessions. Through a series of negotiating sessions, in which a considerable amount of give and take occurs, compromise is eventually reached. As demands are compromised, key contract clauses are developed and a contract begins to take shape. During the negotiating sessions, department heads and supervisors are frequently asked to review specific demands of the union and to present suggestions to higher management. This technique, which utilizes the supervisors' participation, will often bring to light potential problems that may be anticipated in administering the final negotiated contract.

In addition to issues that may have been raised by the union and/or employees during the organizational drive (increased wages, fringe benefits, etc.), the union almost always has vested interests of its own that it introduces as key issues in the negotiating process. First and foremost is the matter of union security, a method of maintaining union membership among the employees.

The union's favored approach is invariably compulsory union membership, commonly known as a "union shop." A typical union shop clause may read:

All present employees who are members of the union (those who signed an authorization card) shall, as a condition of employment, remain members of the union in good standing during the life of this agreement. All employees who at the signing of this agreement are not members of the union must join the union within sixty (60) days of the signing of the agreement. All new hires, after the effective date of the contract, must become members of the union within sixty (60) days from their date of employment and shall as a condition of employment remain members in good standing.

An alternative union security approach is the "maintenance of membership" clause, under which employees who have joined the union must remain as members, but those who are not already members need not join.

A third approach to union security is the "agency shop" agreement, under which employees have the choice of becoming union members and paying dues, or of not joining the union but paying a "fee." Depending on the contract, this fee might be payable to the union or to a designated charity.

A special provision of the amendments to the NLRA also permits an employee of a health care institution who has religious convictions against joining or financially assisting unions to contribute sums equal to any required union dues or fees to one of three nonreligious charitable funds listed in a health care institution's bargaining contract, or to such a fund of his choice if the contract fails to list nonreligious charitable funds.

Another key union issue is usually dues checkoff, or direct deduction of union dues from members' paychecks. Much more important to the union than to the employer, this clause is usually included in contracts, often in exchange for a provision sought by management.

After negotiation and development of the basic issues, such as hours of work, definition of overtime, holiday pay, vacation pay, pension plans, and health and life insurance, attention usually turns to the weight to be given to employee seniority. This will include the questions of how seniority will affect transfers, promotions, decreases or increases in the workforce, and so on. Attention will also be paid to which type of seniority (e.g., employment seniority, department seniority, position seniority, etc.) will be relevant to each type of decision.

Management, too, will have its key issues. Among management's concerns are the no-strike clause and the issue of "management rights."

A management rights clause defines the areas of authority reserved for management: the rights to direct the workforce, to hire, to transfer workers, to set work rules; to decide position qualifications; to purchase or change equipment, and so on. Although most arbitrators take the position that all management rights not limited by the contract definitionally remain in effect, a strong management rights clause is still a potent tool for handling grievances or presenting cases at arbitration.

The no-strike clause is also one of management's most important issues, particularly in the health care field, where an interruption of work could seriously affect patient safety. Of course, a no-strike agreement will be enforceable only during the period of the contract itself; it has no effect after a contract has expired or before an initial contract has been negotiated.

However, to minimize work stoppages at health care institutions and provide continuity of patient care, Congress wrote into the NLRA a new restriction that prohibits a labor organization from striking or picketing a health care institution, or engaging in any other concerted refusal of work, without first giving the employer and the Federal Mediation and Conciliation Service (FMCS) a 10-day written notice of such action. The section specifies, "The notice shall state the date and time that such action will commence. The notice, once given, may be extended by the written agreement of both parties."[1]

This provision will obviously help management plan for a possible strike scenario. However, it is imperative that management, in the initial collective bargaining process, secure a firm contract provision that under no circumstances will there be a work stoppage or slowdown during the life of the contract itself. Moreover, management should be aware that no-strike agreements may be held to apply only to disputes over arbitrable issues, unless drafted in a manner that is clearly intended to encompass *all* possible strikes occurring during the contract term.

The health care amendments to the NLRA also call for special contract renewal/changes and dispute-settling provisions. A 90-day written notice must be served by the employer or union of intent to terminate or modify a collective bargaining contract. If a dispute is involved and indications are that it will continue, the FMCS and appropriate state agencies must be given at least 60 days notice; if a dispute arises in bargaining for an initial contract, at least 30 days' notice must be given by the union to the employer, FMCS, and the appropriate state agencies. The FMCS is empowered to compel the parties to submit to conciliation and dispute resolution, including, at the agency's option, a mandatory period of fact-finding, with public recommendations of settlement by the fact-finding board. All else failing, the 10-day strike or picketing notice must still be served.

Once a union has won certification, the negotiating process has been completed, and a contract has been agreed to, attention must be directed to living with the new rules of the workplace. The new rules imposed by the union contract will govern many, if not all, management-employee relationships. In addition, supervisors and department heads will have a new challenge in controlling their departments. In the nonunion setting, supervisors' authority is rarely challenged or questioned; they have a free hand in dealing with employee relations problems, setting up work schedules, disciplining employees, and the like.

In a unionized facility, this is no longer the case. Once a contract is signed, the shop steward (an employee selected by other employees in the department to act as their spokesperson in grievances and disciplinary proceedings) will pose a constant challenge to the supervisor's authority.

The shop steward represents the union to the employees. As the person who defends the employee against alleged unfair actions of management, he or she is, in fact, the essence of the union to the employees. Unless the supervisor is willing to abdicate responsibility for running the department to the shop steward, or to engage in a long period of unproductive hostility, he or she will recognize an immediate need to develop a spirit of mutual respect, cooperation, and coexistence with the steward.

Shop stewards are frequently the most ardent and vocal supporters of the union among the employees. They receive many hours of education and training by the union; they are completely knowledgeable of all phases of the negotiated contract and know the extent and breadth of management's authority under a contract. But above all, they learn how to deal with the front-line supervisor.

The steward occupies the same position within the union organization as the supervisor does in the organizational structure. Therefore, the relationship between the supervisor and the shop steward will determine to a great extent the severity of future labor-management problems. Supervisors vary in attitude and temperament, but they all must develop the understanding that the union is the authorized representative of the employee. Similarly, the steward must acknowledge the supervisor's authority and responsibility that the supervisor has for operating the department. The need for mutual understanding between supervisor and steward of respective roles and responsibilities cannot be overstressed.

Employees covered by a collective bargaining agreement almost always have at their disposal an appeal process to use when they feel they have been treated unjustly or when a contract provision has been violated. This is, of course, the contractual grievance procedure. Most of us are familiar with grievance procedures, but the picture becomes somewhat clouded in the unionized situation. Now the employee is helped in the formulation, presentation, and appeal of his grievance by the shop steward and the union.

Grievance handling by management in the unionized facility should follow the same procedures as in any well-run workplace. The first action should be the investigation of the grievance and not a prejudgment of its validity. The timeframe in which the grievance is answered is also critical, and efforts should be made for the prompt adjustment of any grievance. Usually the contract will have a defined grievance procedure with a definite timetable, and management is well advised to minimize grievance deadlines and to press for a clause providing that failure to process a grievance in timely fashion renders it waived. (The chart in Exhibit 10-1 shows one possible flow of a grievance in a unionized institution.)

Generally, the last step in any grievance procedure contained in a collective bargaining agreement is grievance arbitration. Thus, when the union and the facility are unable to resolve by mutual agreement a dispute arising from contract interpretation or application, the dispute is submitted to an impartial third party for resolution, often through the auspices of an arbitration agency. The solution reached is final and binding on both the institution and the union, provided that the arbitrator has not exceeded his authority under the contract.

In a nonunion institution, discipline and discharge of an employee is an understood management right, subject only to various state and federal statutes, and to an increasing body of "wrongful discharge" decisions by state courts. However, in the unionized facility, the collective bargaining agreement imposes clear limits on management's disciplinary powers. While these limitations do not prohibit management's right to discipline its employees, the burden of proof now lies with management to provide sufficient and appropriate reasons for discipline and discharge. Almost always, for example, the contract will provide that discharge or discipline must be for "just cause." In addition, discipline or discharge proceedings may be accompanied by and based upon a contractual due process provision that gives employees the opportunity to defend their actions.

Despite the limitations and the need for due process under the mechanisms of the collective bargaining agreement, it would behoove us to recognize that

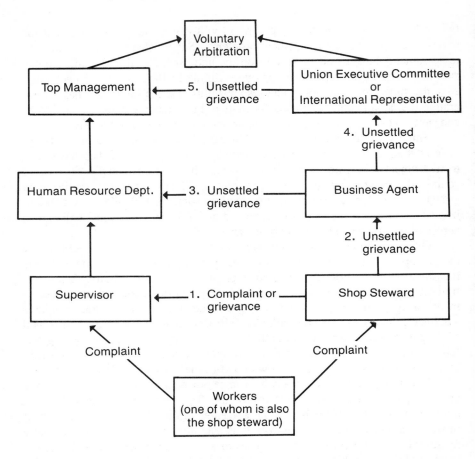

Exhibit 10-1. Grievance procedure in a unionized facility. Note the points at which the union can take an unsettled grievance to higher management.

these clauses usually represent protective rights that should be extended to employees whether a union exists or not. Institutions must develop uniform application and enforcement of work rules and personnel policies. A procedure of progressive discipline should be adopted, including such items as a verbal warning, written warnings, (both containing remedial action, if necessary), employee comments, and penalty for repeated violations, while leaving the employer with enough flexibility to respond to unique employee disciplinary problems.

Sharing control of a facility with a union, especially when it results from a long, hard-fought campaign, may not be the most desirable situation from a management perspective. However, with mutual respect and understanding between administration and union, living with a negotiated contract can be less painful. An attitude must be developed in which the well-being of patients and the concerns of employees, the union, and administration are all respected, understood and balanced.

DIFFICULTIES SUPERVISORS HAVE IN DEALING WITH UNIONIZED EMPLOYEES

Upper management must realize that the front-line supervisors are neither union members nor members of upper management and, as such, they need a lot of management support to maintain a level of authority in a unionized facility. Some of the difficulties they encounter with unionized employees are:

- **Insubordination.** Some newly unionized employees feel that they are beyond the control of the supervisor and challenge authority at every opportunity.

- **Unauthorized or chronic absenteeism.** A few employees attempt to use their shop steward to sanction all of their absences.

- **Substandard performance.** Supervisors may have a difficult time proving that some employees are not meeting the standards for the job because of imprecise contract language.

- **Employee complaints.** Employees frequently misread contract language and complain to the supervisor or the shop steward about their perceived "grievances."

- **Sustaining disciplinary action.** Disciplinary actions are occasionally appealed to outside arbitration, where a neutral third party judges the appropriateness of the supervisor's action(s). Sometimes the decision will favor the employee, and the reversal will be difficult for the supervisor to accept.

- **Assignment of work.** Supervisors have to review contract provisions before assigning new types of tasks to unionized workers.

- **Policies and procedures.** Sometimes the institution will develop new rules and policies that may run counter to the provisions of the union contract. Supervisors must check every new policy and procedure against the negotiated contract and, if they differ, modify the policy/procedure to coincide with the union contract.

HOW MANAGEMENT CAN PROVIDE SUPPORT TO SUPERVISORS

Supervisors in a unionized facility must call on all of their management skills in managing their departments. They must be able to handle grievances, wisely allocate distribution of work, communicate often and accurately, make sound judgments, and above all have a lot of patience. The following guidelines may be helpful to top management in providing support to the front line supervisors:

- Understand and realize that unions frequently divide the loyalty of employees between supervisors and unions. The major concern that supervisors have is that departmental labor problems will reflect adversely on their ability to manage.

- Recognize that administering agreements is time-consuming. The collective bargaining process involves two major phases--first, the negotiation of the agreement, and second, its administration, that is, making it work on a day-to-day basis. Of the two phases, the last one is by far the most time-consuming. Supervisors, therefore, should be given assistance if needed in order for them to be able to devote some time to the administration aspects of the agreement.

- Communicate frequently with supervisors. They need to know that they have upper management's support and confidence, and that being overruled on a grievance does not represent a loss of that support.

- Be knowledgeable. Keep up with developments in labor law and labor relations in order to alert supervisors of changes taking place and to give them factual and current advice.

THE ARBITRATION PROCESS

"Arbitration is the reference of a dispute, by voluntary agreement of the parties, to an impartial person for determination on the basis of evidence and arguments presented by such parties, who agree in advance to accept the decisions of the arbitrator as final and binding."[2]

There are basically two types of arbitration in labor relations: "grievance arbitration" and "interest arbitration." We have touched on grievance arbitration above, in the context of resolving employee or union allegations that the employer has violated the collective bargaining agreement.

Far less common is interest arbitration, in which the independent arbitrator is actually called upon to determine what should be in the contract itself. For example, a contract may provide that if jobs are substantially changed by management, a new wage rate will be determined by agreement between the employer and the union. Failing such agreement, the contract may provide for interest arbitration, in which the parties argue their cases to an arbitrator, who is empowered to decide what the new contract rate will be. On rare occasions, parties negotiating a new contract may even agree to allow unresolved noneconomic issues to be settled via interest arbitration, to eliminate the possibility of a costly and disruptive strike scenario.

PROFESSIONALISM VS. COLLECTIVE BARGAINING

The question of professionalism versus collective bargaining has been debated and disputed. Is professionalism compatible with collective bargaining? Should registered nurses, pharmacists, interns, physical therapists, social workers, laboratory technologists, etc., belong to a union, particularly if this brings prospects of work stoppages, picketing, and other job actions traditional to labor unions?

In education, the question of professionalism versus collective bargaining is not a prominent issue. More than 56 percent of public school teachers are union members. Also, the National Education Association (NEA) has approximately 1.7 million members; the rival American Federation of Teachers (AFT) has approximately 500,000 members. More than 500 colleges and universities have collective bargaining contracts covering 141,000 faculty and professional staff.[3]

In the health care industry, collective bargaining agreements are common for interns working in New York, Chicago, and Los Angeles. The interns are represented by the Physicians National Housestaff Association (PNHA), which represents about 2/3 of the country's 60,000 interns and residents.[4] Other physicians, particularly those who have acquired salaried employee status in hospitals, have followed the route of the interns and gone to collective bargaining. The American Nurses Association (ANA) represents more than 100,000 nurses through its state affiliates.[5] Other unions pursuing health care professionals for collective bargaining purposes are the American Federation of Teachers, District 1199 of the National Union of Hospital and Health Care Employees, the Service Employees International Union, the United Food and Commercial Workers Union, and the Teamsters.

Thus, it appears that the clash between professionalism and collective bargaining has been resolved, and the question has been answered on the positive side of collective bargaining. It is now an accepted fact that all workers, professional and nonprofessional alike, are equally concerned with their economic security, welfare, and working conditions.

Still, many health care workers continue to view the collective bargaining process as a last resort for resolving long-standing issues of concern. Experience has shown that employees will not seek the collective bargaining process when an effective human resource program is in effect. This remains true for both professional and nonprofessional health care workers.

ENDNOTES

1. Labor Management Act of 1947, also known as the Taft-Hartley Act, Section 213, which covers Conciliation of Labor Disputes in the Health Care Industry.

2. Norman Metzger and Joseph M. Ferentino, *The Arbitration and Grievance Process*. Rockville, Maryland: Aspen Publication, 1983.

3. Joseph W. Garbarino and John Lawler, "Faculty Union Activity in Higher Education: 1978," *Industrial Relations* 18 (Spring 1979):244-246.

4. American Hospital Association, *Taft-Hartley Amendments: Implications for the Health Care Field* (Chicago 1976: p. 55).

5. "An Open Letter to the Nurses of America," *American Journal of Nursing* 80 (January 1980):61; reprinted in *AORN Journal* 31 (March 1980): 718-720.

CHAPTER 11

Preparing to Renegotiate the Labor Contract

The best time to prepare for the renegotiation of a labor contract is the instant the contract is ratified and implemented. Therefore, sensitivity should be maintained during the process of presenting the new labor contract to the management and supervisory staff responsible for the implementation of the agreement to detect areas of concern, anxiety, and disappointment. Each of these areas should be identified and discussed, and some record retained by which to either discredit or verify the concern and to identify specific issues that require modification or deletion in subsequent negotiations. Before the impact of the actual negotiations is dissipated, members of the negotiating committee should jointly review their own notes, compare the resulting agreement with their expectations, and itemize areas of concern.

PREPARATION FOR RENEGOTIATIONS

The new agreement should be separated into a clause book so that each article or major clause is on a separate page. This permits notes to be retained regarding how the union used that particular clause, how management interpreted it, and what difficulties it has created for management during the implementation year. It is strongly suggested that each supervisory manager who has to live with the agreement have such a clause book. At the end of the contract prior to renegotiations, each supervisor should prepare a summary of what he or she wants deleted, modified, or inserted by so indicating on the notes. All such clause books should be collected and reviewed by the negotiating committee in establishing strategy for renegotiations.

Since the union sells itself to the membership based on the mistakes that management has made during the contract year, it seems important for management to review its own operational practices with regard to the bargaining unit. It should try to come up with lists of possible deficiencies from the points of view of not only supervisory management or administration but also of a member of the bargaining unit--which should give some idea of what to expect in the way of demands.

THE NEED FOR A BASIC FRAMEWORK

Prior to negotiating any labor agreement, management negotiators should have a firm philosophy to guide the formulation of their proposals and their positions on the union proposals. For instance, the collective bargaining agreement must:

- be consistent with the operational philosophy of the health care facility
- be administratively possible
- preserve management's right to manage the business.

The old agreement ought to be checked against these three considerations, but certainly any new agreement should be challenged by management from those three points of view before reaching final agreement, particularly if there are clauses in the old agreement that:

- adversely affect efficiency
- unduly restrict the right of management to act
- are costly to the institution
- result in excessive grievance
- are vague or ambiguous.

If any such clauses are uncovered, proposals to correct the situation should be drafted. It is also important that the agreement protect internal equity. Has provision been made under the agreement to disproportionately benefit or penalize members of the bargaining unit in any way that would create inequity among employees or employee groups? Is external competition in any way jeopardized by the agreement? Are working conditions such that management can recruit and retain the necessary staff and also protect the patients? Is the facility competitive in terms of services that can be provided and prices that must be charged in order to live with the contract?

LIMITING THE SCOPE OF NEGOTIATIONS

To a large extent the philosophy to be used during the collective bargaining renegotiations may determine the demands that might be presented. Management can put its best foot forward in making its own position clear, fully supportable, and based on NLRB and/or court decisions. Management cannot present a "take it or leave it" position. The general approach should be to make a demand that permits bargaining room. If management fails to make any proposal, it will be assumed that the conditions in the present contract are the base against which management will bargain. It might be to management's advantage to determine specific positions providing less than the existing agreement (perhaps reflecting conditions in previous agreements that were generally satisfactory), which could then counter the extreme position that may be requested by the union. Too often the union presents its premediation position as one of having yielded to management's pressure, when all the union has actually done is move from unrealistic, excessive demands to a position of liberal realism.

Several other factors need to be considered prior to the first negotiation meeting:

- Review the present agreement to separate those articles, clauses, sections, and even sentences that should be retained as well as those that should be eliminated.

- Identify articles, clauses, sections or even sentences that should be modified or changed and designate word, punctuation, or substantive changes desired.

- Direct special attention to any burdensome responsibility that the agreement places on management.

- In terms of the health care facility's short-range and long-term plans, what rights must be retained by management so that the contract does not become a deterrent or an inhibiting factor in future program implementation?

MEDIATION AND ARBITRATION

The 1974 health care amendments added a sentence to section 8(d) of the NLRA that modifies the notice provisions of section 8(d) whenever the collective bargaining involves employees of a health care institution. Thus a party desiring to terminate or modify a labor agreement involving employees of a health care institution must serve written notice of such intention upon the other party 90 (instead of 60) days prior to the actual or proposed termination or modification.[1]

Section 8(d)(1) of the 1974 amendments, if read literally, appears to alter the requirements to notify the Federal Mediation and Conciliation Service (FMCS). Prior to the 1974 amendments, section 8(d)(3) provided that the party desiring termination or modification should notify the FMCS and any state agency established to mandate and conciliate disputes within 30 days after notice to the other party. Section 8(d)(1) of the 1974 amendments provides that "the notice of section 8(d)(3) shall be 60 days."[1] It seems to be generally accepted that this is an error in the 1974 amendments and that notice to the FMCS is actually required within 30 days of the notice to the other party or 60 days prior to the proposed termination or modification.[2] No court has actually stated that there was a drafting error, but two courts have said there appears to have been one. *Sinai Hospital of Baltimore, Inc. v. Scearce*, 561 F. 2d 547, 549 (4th Cir. 1977), *Affiliated Hospitals of San Francisco v. Scearce*, 583 F. 2d 1097, 1098 (9th Cir. 1978).[1]

Section 8(d)(1) of the 1974 amendments also added a special requirement providing that where the bargaining is for an initial agreement following certification or recognition, at least 30 days' notice of the existence of a dispute must be given by the labor organization to the agencies set forth in section 8(d)(3), i.e., to the FMCS and to any state agency established to mediate and conciliate disputes, before a 10-day strike notice can be given.

Mandatory Mediation

Section 8(d)(1) of the 1974 amendments also added a provision to section 8(d) of the NLRA that states that after notice is given, the FMCS shall promptly communicate with the parties and use its best efforts, by mediation and conciliation, to bring them to agreement. It also provides that the parties shall participate fully and promptly in such meetings as may be undertaken by the FMCS for the purpose of aiding in a settlement of the dispute.

Board of Inquiry

The 1974 amendments added section 213 to the NLRA to provide for a board of inquiry. The amendment states that if in the opinion of the FMCS director a threatened or actual strike or lockout affecting a health care institution will substantially interrupt the health care delivery in the locality, the director may establish within 30 days after the notice to the FMCS an impartial board of inquiry to investigate the disputed issues and make a written report to the parties within 15 days after establishing the board. The report must contain findings of fact and recommendations for settling the dispute in a prompt, peaceful, and just way. The board may have as many members as the director wants, as long as none of them has any interest or involvement in the health care institutions or the employee organizations involved in the dispute. After the board is established and for 15 days after it issues the report, there can be no change in the status quo in effect prior to the expiration of the contract in the case of negotiations for a contract renewal, or in effect prior to the time of impasse in the case of an initial bargaining negotiation, unless the parties agree otherwise.

On July 20, 1979, the FMCS promulgated regulations that provide an optional procedure for submitting to the FMCS a list of suggested arbitrators or other individuals who would be acceptable to both the employer and the union as board of inquiry members. The FMCS can defer to the parties' own privately agreed-to fact finding and decline to appoint a Board of Inquiry so long as the parties' procedure meets certain conditions that are set forth in the regulations and satisfy the responsibilities of the FMCS under the NLRA.

Collective bargaining is a dynamic and fluid process that places a premium on flexibility, ingenuity, and patience; the challenge confronting negotiators is immense. In collective bargaining, as in so many other endeavors, there is no substitute for thorough preparation. It cannot be stressed too much that collective bargaining is a two-way street, and that there is a continued need during the negotiation process for sound judgment and supportable fact to establish and maintain a strong position. There is truth in the old statement that a job well begun is half done.

EMERGENCY ARRANGEMENTS

There is almost an infinite variety of strategic and tactical approaches that can be pursued in negotiating a labor contract. Strategies and tactics will vary as the facts change.

Management should always bargain in good faith but also accept that every once in a while the best organized plans will go askew. Strikes or other forms of work interruptions should always be considered a possibility. Since the likelihood of these emergency situations appears to be increasing in the health care field, health care facilities should develop emergency arrangements for dealing with all types of work interruptions. Such arrangements are the topic of the next chapter.

ENDNOTES

1. Labor Management Act of 1947, also known as the Taft-Hartley Act of 1947.

2. Marshall B. Babson, Jeanette C. Schreiber. *Issues Arising Under the 1974 Health Care Amendments to the National Labor Relations Act*, pp. 51-54. Wiggin and Dana Counsellors at Law, New Haven, Conn., 1984.

CHAPTER 12

Planning for Work Stoppages

The American Nurses' Association distributes to its member associations various pamphlets on how to engage in a successful strike. These pamphlets usually stress that prior to engaging in a strike, employees need to assess their strength, a philosophy that is held by all unions. The premise is not to engage in a work stoppage that they are going to lose.

No health care facility likes even to think about service disruptions resulting from union contract negotiations. It is a fact of life, however, that needs to be addressed since the ultimate union weapon is the strike call. Health care facilities that are prepared to deal with all kinds of work stoppages, with all contingencies, will most likely survive any crisis with as few inconveniences as possible to their patients, services, facilities, staff, and, of course, the community. Therefore, an effective strike plan established by the health care facility can serve as a deterrent for unions to decide, after assessing their power, that it is better to settle than to strike. There can come a point during the collective bargaining process when collective bargaining options appear closed and a strike appears unavoidable.

Unless an assessment has been made of the health care facility's ability to take a strike, the facility may find itself in a precarious situation. Running a health care facility during a work stoppage demands punctilious advance planning; even so, it is one of the most stressful experiences managers will ever have to deal with during their professional careers.

The NLRA requires that a labor organization give a 10-day notice to a health care institution prior to a strike. Although health care facilities have this 10-day advance notice to prepare for a work stoppage, they should not wait until that time to decide how they will operate during the strike. Exhibit 12-1 depicts a summarized example of a strike plan.

```
XYZ HEALTH CARE

SUBJECT:  Strike Preparation Plan
POLICY & PROCEDURE NO.   90-3

(SPP)  (May also be used                 Effective Date:  3/4/80
for any other type of work               Revised:  5/85
interruption)                            Reviewed:  January, 1986

DEPARTMENT RESPONSIBLE:  PERSONNEL

AUTHORIZATION:
                                         _____
                                         Department Head(s)
                                         Committee Chairman
                        (or)             Management Team member
                        (or)             Chief of Staff
                        (or)             President
```

Exhibit 12-1.

I. PURPOSE

On the premise that labor organizations--both unions and professional associations--can, will and do strike health care facilities despite the implications on responsible care of the sick, the following outline is an operational plan designed to protect the welfare and best interest of our patients in the event of an anticipated or sudden work interruption situation. This plan can also be used for any other work interruptions not necessarily related to a labor dispute.

II. POLICY

To maintain at all times an operational plan and basic course of action to be followed in the event XYZ Health Care should experience any work interruption incidents within any or all of its departments or units. This policy outlines the general guidelines to be followed; the contents may be altered if it is determined that the welfare of XYZ, patients, or fellow employees require it.

III. RESPONSIBILITY

The Strike Preparation Plan (SPP) outlines a basic description of the activities and responsibilities of several departments whose operational functions will become paramount in the event of a work interruption incident. ALL DEPARTMENTS SHOULD REVIEW THESE OUTLINES AND DEVELOP SPECIFIC TANDEM PLANS FOR THEIR AREAS. The president of XYZ shall be the Strike Plan leader (SPL). The alternate SPL shall be in order, the vice-president--operations, the vice-president--personnel and employee relations, and the vice-president--finance. It will be the SPL's responsibility to activate the provisions of this policy. The decision to activate the SPP will be made in consultation with the management team members. This group will maintain 24-hour/7-day per week coverage of the administration offices. It will be the responsibility of the management team to phase into operation, as needed, departments and/or functions under their jurisdiction. The management team members will also be responsible for maintaining daily communications with their department heads relative to the status of work interruption incident. As needed, any members of management may be assigned on a temporary basis to other duties in any area of the institution.

IV. PROCEDURE

A. *Personnel Needs*

Management team members will assess the personnel needs for each area affected. The procedure will be:

Exhibit 12-1, cont.

Step 1 An evaluation will be made by the management team as to what areas are deficient in qualified personnel.

Step 2 A staff skills inventory will be taken in each department of employees *not involved in the work stoppage*. Forms are available through the vice-president--personnel and employee relations.

Step 3 The management team using the staff skills inventory will match personnel to assignments and will inform the individuals concerned of their SPP assignments.

Step 4 The director of education will immediately implement emergency training programs to fill the requirements for areas still in need of specific talents. Individuals from any area of the facility may be considered/selected for these skill development training programs.

Step 5 The director of volunteer services will conduct an audit of volunteer skills. The information obtained by means of this audit will assist in assigning volunteers to tasks they can perform most effectively. Additional support from the community will be elicited as needed. The director of volunteer services, the president, the labor relations counsel, the vice-president-- personnel and employee relations, and the vice-president--nursing affairs will meet for guidance in determining the role and activities of volunteers during the work interruption.

Step 6 The SPL will initiate all support actions by contacting the appropriate health care association and various health care institutions in the areas.

Step 7 The SPL will notify the chiefs of the clinical services that the SPP is being implemented and that a reduction of the census to a manageable level will be necessary.

Step 8 Depending on the extent of the situation, a directive may be issued by the SPL to all employees of the XYZ stating that days off for nonemergency leaves, vacations and/or holidays will be suspended during the period of SPP.

Exhibit 12-1, cont.

B. Medical Staff Assistance

In the event of a work stoppage, the SPL will consult with the Medical Staff on areas needing their support.

C. Operational Needs

1. *Reduction of Census*

Within four hours of the implementation of the SPP, the medical staff in the respective services should submit plans regarding the disposition of their patients to their chiefs of service. A combined list of the disposition plans for all patients on the particular service will be forwarded to the admitting office, the social service department and the management team. All patients who can be safely discharged will be sent home if their personal physicians approve the discharge. Names of patients who need assistance at home will be given to the management team for possible assistance by community members who will be enlisted on a volunteer basis to assist in certain patient care functions such as feeding, bathing, etc. Members of the management team will make arrangements with other facilities, regional health agencies, public health nursing and nursing homes for those patients requiring skilled nursing care within the institution.

Admitting will maintain information pertaining to where patients are sent. As the census decreases, admitting, with the cooperation and aid of the nursing office, will begin to consolidate the patients on the nursing units, as well as by buildings.

2. *Admissions*

The admitting office will continue to admit emergency patients and make in-house transfers. Limited inpatient capacity will be the immediate and anticipated short-range goal of the SPP; therefore, it is imperative that admissions be on a priority basis. The priority requisites will be reviewed on an individual basis by the chief of the medical staff.

3. *Dietary Services*

Dietary services for patients will be the first priority during the SPP. Food services for facility personnel may be curtailed entirely or limited to continental breakfast, sandwiches, soup and drinks for lunch and supper meal depending on the extent of the work interruption. All special function caterings may be suspended. Plastic/paper dishes will be used for

Exhibit 12-1, cont.

patient/employee meals, etc., depending on the
extent of the situation.
 Meals supplied under the SPP will be kept as
simple and easy to prepare as possible.
Selective menus will not be available.
Convenience foods and canned vegetables instead
of frozen vegetables will be used. Inventory
levels should be increased so that a four (4)
week supply of food items and nonfood items are
on hand.

4. *Housekeeping Services*

Housekeeping services for patient rooms, patient
care areas, and the dietary department will be
given priority over all other areas.
Housekeeping services for offices, waiting rooms,
corridors, elevators, etc., will be on a rotating
weekly, as-needed, basis.

5. *Laundry Services*

The materials manager will immediately assess the
laundry needs for areas in operation during the
SPP and determine if laundry capabilities will be
adequate. The extensive use of disposables will
be considered and arrangements made for outside
laundry services as needed. Production and/or
distribution of uniforms, lab coats, smocks,
etc., will be on a limited basis as needed.

6. *Security Services*

Continuation of the security functions will be
maintained in order to provide adequate property
protection, fire rounds, and a fire brigade in
the event of an emergency. As needed, additional
private police will be engaged to augment the
current staff to maximize security. Security
services will be utilized to provide protection
of vital supplies as well as to assist employees
leaving or reporting for work.

7. *Public Relations*

Understandably, during a work interruption the
patients and their families will be extremely
apprehensive. They will need reassurance that
the institution is fully capable of maintaining a
high level of patient care. The director--
corporate communications will assume all public
communication responsibilities during a work
interruption incident. Letters will be sent to
families of patients as soon as possible.
Similarly, prospective patients who have been
scheduled for admission will be informed as soon
as possible of any difficulties that might be
occasioned by the work interruption. During the
first several days, public/press interest is apt

Exhibit 12-1, cont.

to be high. If conditions warrant it or there is anticipation of operational difficulties with press information overtones, it may be necessary for the corporate communications office to work a 12-hour day from 8:00 a.m. to 8:00 p.m., including weekends.

8. *Communications*

Routine staffing at each switchboard should be adequate; however, the director of communications should closely supervise each shift to assure that public/press inquiries on the work interruption are channeled to the corporate communications office. If necessary, an answering device with a taped message should be attached to an extension referring general inquiries to an outside number(s) at which public relations personnel can be reached.

9. *Pharmacy*

The pharmacy's vital function during the SPP will consist of filling inpatient prescription orders, providing floor stock drugs, and delivering IV solutions. Employee prescription orders will be suspended during the SPP. The director of pharmacy services shall have the option to request that OPD and ER prescriptions be filled in community pharmacies if the work load becomes greater than can be managed by available personnel. Levels of pharmaceuticals should be increased so that an ample four-week supply is on hand.

10. *Nursing Service*

The nursing department will be *the* central function of XYZ at all times during a work interruption situation, and its continued performance will be the most important activity to be covered in the event the SPP is activated. Every effort will be made to concentrate the sickest patients remaining in the facility in areas with the highest nursing staff and the greatest amount of emergency equipment. Beyond the use of the OB/CCU/ICU/PAR/OR, any seriously ill patients should be grouped into 2- or 4-bed rooms, where possible, and assigned adequate nursing staff to cover the 2 or 4 beds on a 24-hour basis. All nursing service personnel (full- and part-time) may be required to work more than their regular scheduled hours.

11. *Materials Management*

In the event the SPP is activated, the materials management director will ascertain that inventory levels are maintained so that XYZ will have a

Exhibit 12-1, cont.

four-week supply of critical items on hand at all times. The inventory review will also take into consideration the plan for the dietary department to use plastic and paper dishes to serve patient and employee meals, and additional linen for the laundry department. Extensive use of disposables will be stressed. To assure that XYZ receives deliveries and essential supplies, the director of materials management will contact regular common carriers or major suppliers to ascertain that deliveries will be made. If necessary, XYZ will rent trucks and supply drivers to pick up essential materials. Arrangements may also be made for suppliers to deliver cargo to an off-campus warehouse.

12. *Data Processing*

The data processing director shall provide and/or make arrangements to provide special protection for XYZ's data bank systems, important records or documents.

13. *Plant Operations and Engineering*

With professional security counsel, the director of plant operations will determine means by which vital equipment items can be protected against vandalism, identify where equipment should be stored, how protected, and who has access to it. In addition, the director of plant operations shall assure that repairs and maintenance services for vital and critical equipment have priority over all other tasks.

14. *All Other Departments*

During a work interruption the majority of departments not directly affected or involved will function as best as possible on a limited service basis with the managerial staff constantly reviewing their personnel needs and releasing as many employees as possible for utilization in areas affected or directly involved in the work interruption.

V. FILING INSTRUCTIONS

This policy shall be filed in Section 90 of the Policy and Procedures Manual.

VI. DISTRIBUTION

This policy is to be distributed to all departments.

Exhibit 12-1, cont.

STAFF SKILLS INVENTORY

Prepared by: _____

Date: _____

Name	Position title	Other skills, Licenses, certifications, etc.	Possible mobility to:	Emergency trng. required	Area & date assigned

WORK STOPPAGE PREPARATION PLAN

On the premise that labor organizations--both unions and professional associations--can, will, and do strike health care facilities despite the implications for responsible care of the sick, the following outline constitutes specific elements of a strike preparation plan.

I. Objectives
   A. To secure and protect the following:
      1. People
         a. Inpatients
         b. Outpatients
         c. Students
         d. Volunteers
         e. Visitors
         f. Employees
         g. Medical Staff
      2. Facilities
      3. Vital equipment
      4. Vital supplies
      5. Data, records and documentation
      6. Institution image and reputation
   B. To assure in the long-range interest of the institution's position that an unprovoked strike can be successfully withstood by the health care facility with a minimum negative impact and a minimum of compromises that might be necessitated in the face-saving process of strike termination.
   C. To promote positive information flow both internally and externally and to establish and maintain an effective relationship with media.

II. Essential Preparatory Steps:
   A. The health care facility's position, stated in writing, relative to the work stoppage.
   B. The appointment of a command person with specific authority to assume the responsibility for execution of the position.
   C. The establishment of a communication center for information flow to the press as well as for internal and external information.
   D. The identification of individuals who must be called back to the facility/department in the event of a difficult situation.
   E. Development of a specific procedure or action plan to be followed.

III. Positive Posture and Relationship with the Media
   A. Make personal contacts with key individuals representing newspapers, radio, and television, briefly outlining the facility's position and the intent to be cooperative with information flow.
   B. Where a cooperative press relationship is not possible, consider the use of paid advertising as a means of getting the facility's complete message to the public.
   C. Attempt to provide facility staff with advanced copies of information that they can expect to see in the press.
   D. If present staff lacks sufficient time, experience, or qualifications to undertake a positive public relations effort, utilize professional personnel for this responsibility.

IV. Minimize patient care requirements both to protect the legal responsibilities of the facility and to create a psychological impact on potential strikers that the institution is in readiness. An occupied bed encourages the striker by suggesting that the facility cannot afford to be without personnel. An empty bed will likewise discourage the striker. Consider the following possibilities in sequence.
   A. Discontinue patient admissions approximately four days prior to the strike deadline except for emergency cases.
   B. Arrange with other health care facilities for temporary privileges for medical staff and for possible emergency admissions as early as the day before the strike but definitely on the day of the strike if a strike does materialize.
   C. Through a medical review committee determine several days prior to the strike deadline those patients that could be discharged if necessary without jeopardy to their well-being in the event there is insufficient personnel to meet patient care requirements. Have this list prepared for immediate use if necessary.
   D. In the event of a serious strike and minimal staff, make prior arrangements for the possible transfer of patients the day of the strike if necessary to maintain adequate patient care.
   E. Cancel outpatient service programs and give adequate notice to the public.
   F. Consider the necessity of temporarily closing Emergency Room service and provide for adequate notice to the public.

V. Staffing requirements and availability
   A. Through the supervisors establish a list naming each employee indicating:

1. The employees who can be expected to recognize the strike call and not be on duty.

2. The employees who can be expected to come through the picket lines and be on duty.

3. The employees who would prefer to be on duty but are hesitant to come through the picket lines and therefore cannot be counted on for staffing. It is important to indicate the critical reason the supervisor believes the employee is fearful of reporting on duty.

B. Ascertain maximum expected staffing based on those expected to cross the picket line, and plan for not more than one out of five for those who are fearful to cross the picket line. This latter number can be increased if the institution, prior to the strike, can minimize the critical issues creating employee fear and concern.

C. To indicate maximum available staff, identify possible volunteers and additional personnel who could be made available and would be willing to cross the picket lines. This latter group will require special orientation prior to the strike.

D. Determine maximum patient load that should be considered based on available staff, and for conservative planning reduce this number by 20 percent at least for the initial day or few days of the strike. The health care facility will be given credit in the public eye for taking steps to protect patient care interests. It is also psychologically to the advantage of the facility if, after a strike has commenced, it is able to announce that patients can be and are being admitted.

E. Establish immediate plans for the possible permanent replacement of employees who have engaged in an economic strike.

VI. Provide for and expand the present security force with qualified security guards, preferably experienced in strike-bound activities. Commence the orientation of this group at least five days prior to the strike deadline to provide adequate time to gain professional advice on necessary security of the facilities, equipment and supplies. A strong show of security will indicate to the employees the facility's position of attempting to provide full security and will thus encourage employees otherwise uncertain that they can cross picket lines.

VII. Provide as many means as possible to assist employees in crossing the picket line and in receiving protection. This may include but not be limited to:

A. With available beds due to reduced patient admissions, it is possible to provide for some live-in employees. It is suggested that six hours of work, and six hours off around the clock provides the maximum use of available personnel with a minimum fatigue factor. Assign linens to employees living in. Do not assign a bed since the same bed can be shared, doubling the live-in capacity.

B. Provide security to assist employees in walking through the picket line.

C. Consider a van or a bus to pick up employees at predetermined pickup points (such points can be changed daily to avoid union identification of the areas and possible harassment of employees), and drive the employees through the picket lines.

VIII. Provide for reasonable availability and protection of vital supplies.

A. Have each supervisor provide a list based on normal patient occupancy of each supply item that is vital in the care of the patients and the amount of that supply item that is used. Identify possible options to that supply. This will indicate the minimum quantity of basic vital supply items that must be on hand prior to the strike. The total quantity can be reduced proportionately, based on anticipated reductions in patient admissions. It is suggested, however, that to avoid future difficulties of receiving supply items, efforts be made to provide full supply requirements in the event the hospital can successfully withstand the strike.

B. Give special consideration to certain types of supplies that create difficulties, such as:

1. Bulk goods--55 gallon drums of detergents, chemicals, cleaning materials, disinfectants, alcohol, etc., that are difficult to handle. In addition, bulk package goods such as surgical supplies, cotton goods, and disposable items should be obtained in advance. Further, large usage items such as IV solutions should be placed on inventory.

2. Oxygen use should be determined based on capacity, with arrangements for delivery of a final supply the day before the strike. Additional tanks of oxygen and other gases should be considered. Physical protection of the oxygen tank system is also vital.

3. Food supplies should be provided in adequate quantities with emphasis on quick-preparation foods, dehydrated packaged foods, frozen foods, soups, etc. In addition, alternate sources of meal service should be developed.

4. Fuel may be a potential problem. Be assured that the oil tanks are filled or that the fuel supply system will be adequate.

5. Diagnostic and therapeutic drugs, chemicals, reagents, and materials should be provided for at least the first two weeks. Most of these items can be picked up in personal cars for later use.

6. On the premise that the health care facility maintains a normal three-day linen supply, it is necessary to provide a temporary policy to

minimize linen usage, perhaps by changing beds every other day or dropping the top sheet to bottom sheet, etc. Provision for laundry service is essential. Disposable linens are one option. It is absolutely necessary to provide strict security for clean linen supplies. It is simple to splash a bottle of urine across the linen supply, destroying its usefulness.

7. Sterile packs should be prepared in advance, providing adequate security for the packs as they are processed but keeping pack-preparing personnel that might be on strike away from sterile packs for the final two shifts prior to the commencement of the expected strike. It is simple to run a razor blade down a stack of sterile packs and ruin their usefulness.

IX. Provide adequate protection plus repair and maintenance service for vital and critical equipment.

A. Have supervisors prepare a list of specific equipment items that are essential in maintaining adequate patient care with possible alternates or options that are available.

B. Pursue alternate sources, particularly if this is equipment available to other facilities, to establish accessibility prior to the strike and means of delivery.

C. With professional security counsel, determine means by which vital equipment items can be protected against vandalism. Identify where equipment should be stored, how it will be protected, and who has access to it.

D. Consider special precautions to protect steam lines and valves, oxygen lines and valves, suction lines and valves, hot water lines and valves, fluid waste disposal systems, transformer boxes, and fuse box controls.

X. Provide special protection for data bank systems and important records or documents. Consider but do not limit emphasis to the following:

A. Prepare a duplicate of the computer memory bank.

B. Provide special protection for blueprints, schematic drawings and diagrams.

C. Protect other financial, personnel, and patient records including films.

D. Consider protection against theft, destruction, vandalism, and fire or water damage.

XI. Prepare a system for bulk rubbish removal. Attention should be given to the possible increased rubbish supply due to an increased use of disposable items. Special consideration may need to be directed toward garbage and toward human tissue disposal.

XII. Protect against investigative, disruptive, or harassing techniques such as, but not limited to:

A. Community and church leaders and other persons of influence as concerned citizens who volunteer to resolve the institution's problem with disruptive techniques.

B. Specific press conferences at designated times and places to avoid intermittent, sketchy, incomplete or fragmented reporting. Use prepared press release information.

C. Inspections or intervention by government or social agencies based on charges or challenges by the union that:

1. Unsafe working conditions prevail as a result of the strike, requiring inspections from the Occupational Safety and Health inspectors.

2. Violations of equal pay and other factors of the Wage and Hour Law exist and require inspection by Department of Labor.

3. Under-age employees are working without appropriate employment certificates after reasonable hours or in dangerous areas in order to accommodate for the strike, requiring inspection by appropriate State agencies.

4. Employees are discriminated against in terms of race, age, or sex in order to meet minimum staffing requirements, necessitating investigation by the Equal Employment Opportunity Commission.

5. Cleanliness and basic sanitation is poor due to the shortage of housekeeping personnel, increasing the jeopardy of adequate patient care and requiring inspections by the local health department or other public health officials.

6. Other similar harassing practices, each of which requires time to assist in the inspection process and to provide reports. It is also important to consider legal intervention to minimize such harassment.

XIII. Provide for control of employee discipline with detailed documentation. Supervisors should be alerted to get counsel before exercising strict discipline, particularly suspension or discharge, so as to avoid handing the union a martyr or series of martyrs that might negate internal communication efforts to avoid angering employees leaning to the strike. Emphasis should be placed on careful documentation and consultation.

XIV. Identify, in addition to the medical staff and the auxiliary, others that must be kept informed with regard to all or part of the strike preparation activities of the institution and the impact that such activities have on that group. Support should be sought from the medical staff and auxiliary. Suppliers should be advised of the potential strike so as not to waste time if union drivers would refuse to cross the picket lines. The public should be advised to minimize visiting and a visitor control program should be developed.

XV. Attempt to minimize the strike threat itself by appeals to the employees, which may include but not be limited to:

A. Small group meetings of employees to express the health care facility's concern, to reassure concerning security protections that have been planned, and to clarify the facility's position.

B. Present in written form a factual portrayal of the chronology of the negotiation process, the critical factors of the impasse, and the position of the facility to justify its stance.

C. Provide supervisors with appropriate information and positions so that one-on-one or small groups of supervisors can give adequate encouragement to the employees not to strike and assurance of protection if they cross the picket lines.

D. Attempt to minimize the impact of any union threats to employees concerning excessive fines for union members that cross picket lines and harassment of employees. This should include a system of information with witnesses, and written documentation of such problems for future protection of the facility in legal proceedings and the pursuit of unfair labor practice charges.

E. Appeal to the employees' emotions by indicating that their security is dependent upon a healthy facility, not a strong union. Explain what would need to be gained by the strike in increased benefits to offset the loss of wages for one day, two days, one week, two weeks, etc. Discuss other factors in practical terms and a manner understandable to the average employee, with a final appeal not to strike.

XVI. Assuming that the employees do not strike, preparation should be directed toward other forms of union activity. For each of the following there is need for a clear statement of position, designated person in charge, source of communication and list of call-back personnel and a proceduralized action plan:

A. Peaceful demonstrations
   1. Inside the facility by employees
   2. Inside the facility by outsiders
   3. Outside the facility by employees
   4. Outside the facility by outsiders

B. Disruptive demonstrations
   1. Work slowdowns
   2. Work stoppages
   3. Sit-ins

      4. Massive sick calls

      5. Informational pickets

XVII. Miscellaneous considerations

    A. It is important to schedule all employees on duty for their respective shifts on the day the strike is to begin so as to determine whether the employee is with the facility or with the strike and not to delay this determination for one, two or three additional days. If the strike is successful, extra personnel will be needed. There is also a psychological advantage if strikers see an abundance of employees on duty.

    B. It may be important to cancel vacations, particularly for vital personnel, in the event that associates of such personnel would be anticipated to strike. This prevents the employee from maintaining a position of neutrality, using the vacation as an excuse, rather than making a commitment either to the facility or to the union.

XVIII. Final considerations

    A. Be cautious regarding telephone use. If necessary, provide for a private direct line to bypass the switchboard.

    B. Be cautious of disposing in wastebaskets anything that could be useful to the union.

    C. Be cautious of processing through the print shop or on other duplicating equipment anything of confidential nature, as stencils, plates, masters, and scrap copies can easily be transmitted to the union.

The Boy Scouts of America have the motto "Be Prepared," and it has worked very well for them for many years. In labor relations there is a frequently-used Latin sentence that says, "*Si vis pacem para bellum*"--"If you want peace, prepare for war." The adoption of a work stoppage plan does not imply that management considers a work stoppage imminent or even likely, only that it sees it as a possibility. Health care managers have a responsibility to prepare for possibilities that could adversely affect their ability to provide patient care services.

In the final analysis, management needs to be realistic about its responsibilities to patients, the community, and its employees. A planning process for work stoppages should be a key concern in the operation of every health care organization in the country.

PART III

PERSONNEL PRACTICES FOR THE '80s

INTRODUCTION

PERSONNEL PRACTICES FOR THE '80s

The health care personnel management picture is big and growing bigger. There are new jobs, new work environments, and new methods of delivering health care. The American health care system has essentially become a highly competitive industry, and as a result more and more American health care workers now find themselves working outside of the traditional hospital setting, and in new health care work environments such as homecare services for the community, health maintenance organizations, adult day-care programs, home dialysis programs, long-term care facilities, skilled nursing institutions, emergi-centers, and a multitude of community outpatient clinics.

Personnel management in the American health care industry has generally been the result of pressures, crises, special interest groups, special demands, shortages, availabilities and substitutions. In general, one could say that it has been the result of reacting or responding, not of planning. Therefore, in most health care facilities, the personnel management program resembles a patchwork quilt.

Part III depicts a comprehensive personnel program that can be implemented in any health care facility regardless of size, location, ownership, or function. It also goes into the specifics of how to write and implement personnel policies.

Corporate culture is defined in Part III as "a health care institution's breeding." It is suggested that "having a healthy culture will assist both management and employees to cope with the environmental changes taking place in the American health care system."

In this section of the book, the roles of participative management, morale surveys and common-sense solutions to typical problems are discussed and examined.

The authors have also included a chapter on staff reductions and how to prepare for them, and concluded with a chapter on new horizons and new environments for the American health care industry.

All in all, Part III introduces a comprehensive personnel administration program for dealing with union and nonunion employees.

CHAPTER 13

Content of a Comprehensive Personnel Administration Program

As health care financing continues to experience drastic economic changes, health care facilities are increasingly reexamining their operational and administrative practices. The examinations are resulting in a variety of changes and actions. The consistent emerging theme is that the changes are significantly affecting the role and responsibility of the human resource practitioner. As health care facilities continue to work through difficult economic issues, it is becoming more obvious to chief executive officers and governing boards that an organization's human resource program is crucial to an effective and efficient operation. The dilemma of reduced hospital utilization, plus a price-driven system for payment for institutional care, have clearly focused the need for a prudent resource management system within the American health care industry.

With the new surge of interest in health care personnel management, there has come along almost as a byproduct a mistaken notion that the benefits of sound and realistic personnel management can be achieved while practicing only a part of the total personnel management program. There is evidence of health care facilities putting emphasis on one phase of personnel management and then awaiting the vast results that might be expected from a comprehensive program. Then, when such results are not forthcoming, there is also the tendency to condemn the program of personnel management and its many practices as impractical tools designed for industry and not applicable to the health care field.

This is most unfortunate, because one of the greatest potential aids to more effective management becomes lost, at least temporarily, to the facility's chief executive officer. It has been unfortunate, too, because of the tendency to condemn the whole for the failure of one of its parts, especially as many of the parts are not capable of functioning properly without the support and collaboration of other personnel practices and techniques.

Personnel management is a package of many parts, each working best when working in conjunction with the others, and creating a whole greater than their sum. Personnel management includes a set of principles and a philosophy as well as a specific group of techniques and systems. Its scope envelops the job, the worker, and the work environment. In addition to its economic concerns, it has equal interest in social and psychological matters. Its aim--a simple one--is the satisfaction of mutual needs, the needs of the worker as well as the needs of the employer.

But the fulfillment of this aim will not just happen. It will require the proper functioning of many different personnel management techniques properly integrated, properly understood, and properly evaluated if the health care facility is to enjoy the benefits that it should derive from personnel management. There must be an understanding of 12 essential aspects of health care personnel management, each performing its own purposes and contributing to the better performance of some of the other aspects. The following is a detailed explanation of the essentials in health care personnel management.

- **Personnel management is part of, and not separate from, good basic management.** A review of health care management audits indicates a direct correlation between the quality of basic management and the quality of its personnel management. Where management itself is good, both effective and sound, then the personnel program tends also to be both effective and sound. Conversely, it is unlikely that a realistic personnel program will be functioning in a health care facility that has basically unsound management. The personnel program tends to reflect the general quality of the philosophy and practice of management itself.

  There has been recognition that management accomplishes its objectives through people and not through its own immediate efforts. It has, therefore, an objective of developing these people in such a way that they can become more fully productive. In a sense, it is a secondary goal to the primary objective of management, the achievement of a contented employee doing a satisfying and satisfactory job. This involves three key points:

  First, there is the need for a contented worker who by preference would choose the type of job he or she is doing or hopes to do in the health care environment. The employee is there by choice rather than circumstance.

  Second, this worker must be doing a satisfying job, which means that performance meets basic personal needs. This will include not just economic needs through an adequate wage program but also, to at least some extent, social and psychological needs.

  Third, from management's viewpoint, a satisfactory job reflects performance that meets the standards of quality, quantity, time, cost, and -- where it applies--appearance, as established by management and understood and accepted by the worker.

  Personnel management is the process of bringing together the worker and work, placing both in a proper environment. This environment is more than physical; it must include the social, psychological, and managerial environment as well.

  This process of personnel management, like any other form of management, requires a general objective and goal as well as specific short-term objectives. This plan requires an organization and integration and a control of all phases of personnel activity, to be assured of the eventual achievement of the overall objectives.

There is need, too, to enhance the quality and understanding of management within the health care facility. It is not so often a case of bad management as of a lack of management. Past emphasis on professional preparation and technical training of key personnel has prepared them well for operating level positions, but because of the extent of their education, these personnel have tended to be advanced and promoted into positions of supervision and management. The potential difficulty is that they do not consider themselves management, and often do not function as management, tending to regress to the former activities for which they were so well-prepared. This situation has led to the next point in the total personnel package.

- **Personnel management is the responsibility of the supervisor, not of the personnel director.** This may sound somewhat surprising when we so often believe that a personnel director is employed to perform the personnel management functions. Yet upon careful analysis, we can see that because personnel management is a staff function, it accomplishes its work not directly but indirectly through the work of the supervisors, department heads, and administration. It works best when it counsels, assists, advises, recommends, and in other ways enables the supervisor to better carry out the personnel function with the employees.

  The personnel director does not decide what the job will be, what the specifications for employment are, which applicant will be hired, under what conditions the employee is to be discharged, and which employee gets an increase in pay. Those decisions are most often made by the department heads or the supervisors. We could perhaps say that the personnel director directs a personnel program, whereas the supervisor actually directs the employee. This means that supervisors at all levels of the organization need to be acquainted with the personnel management responsibilities and may require training and development in the ability to perform them. Actually, the personnel program rests on the combined abilities of the supervisors to carry out the personnel functions. The personnel director can be only as successful, through the personnel program, as the individual supervisors are in their personnel relations.

- **The goal is well-defined jobs with carefully matched workers, properly and adequately paid.** At first glance it might almost appear that the essence of personnel management is wrapped up in this particular point. It is an important point, and involves the majority of vital issues, techniques, philosophy, and principles of the personnel administration field. It begins with the job analysis, moves into selection techniques, and concludes with wage administration. Now let us examine these point by point.

First, the job analysis is the basis for information on which most of the additional personnel techniques will be based. Superficial job analyses or general descriptions of activities will produce superficial results. Because job analysis itself is a tool of little value until used, it needs to be comprehensive or multipurpose in its objective. Job analysis in the health care facility where there has been little standardization of job activities in the past should be applied to the work of each worker (actually a position analysis). The analysis becomes a word image of what each worker actually does.

The heart of the analysis is a task-by-task description of what the worker does, how the worker does it, why the worker does this activity in this particular way, how often the activity is performed, what percentage of the total work time is spent in performing it, how difficult the task is (assuming the worker is competent to perform it), what degree of authority the worker has in performing this activity, and what the performance standards are--regarding quality, what quantity, time to complete the work, cost of performance and (where it applies) appearance of the completed work.

This type of detailed, task-by-task analysis enables the personnel director as well as the supervisors and department heads to develop many useful and essential personnel techniques. Very quickly the job or position specification can be ascertained: If the worker is to perform all these tasks in the prescribed way, what types of knowledge, skill, education, and experience must he or she possess? The same job analysis will pinpoint necessary items for orientation to the job. Job instruction is essentially outlined under the conditions regarding how the work is performed. The performance requirements that can easily be developed from the above information will serve as a basis for job evaluation and eventually total wage administration.

Once there is a basic understanding of the job, systematic selection for the worker can begin. The job precedes the worker, and in a sense dictates the kind of worker required if that job is to be properly performed. An understanding of the job, then, enables effective recruitment to begin, looking not just for applicants, but for persons of specific qualifications. A meaningful application blank can record facts about the applicant that can be compared with the specifications of the job. The interview can give depth and meaning to the facts on the application blank as well as open new areas for discussion and mutual understanding. Verification of references and investigation of past performance on other jobs, similar or even unrelated, give further evidence of the potential competence of the applicant to perform the job in question. Testing, too, plays an important part in selection, so that one is not moved on faith but attempts to verify through tests certain areas of knowledge or skill or aptitude that the job may require. A physical examination determines whether the applicant is physically able to do the job in question.

In a sense, systematic selection attempts to find out as much about the applicant as job analysis attempts to find out about the job or work to be performed. The final choice as to which applicant will be employed is a matter of matching the job specifications with the worker's qualifications. When there is a match and also an appropriate social and psychological base on which to fit the applicant into the department, then proper selection becomes possible.

Selection, however, does not finish the process of bringing the worker onto the job. Once the decision has been made, the person needs to be oriented to the health care facility, to the department, and to the job.

Orientation to the facility is simply an introduction: What is it? How is it unique? How is it different? Why is it important? What are the advantages of this type of employment?

The department needs a similar introduction. The applicant may have been placed in the housekeeping department, or dietary, or clerical work, or perhaps in nursing service. Each is unique, and the worker should appreciate the particular importance of the department to which he or she has been assigned and how it contributes to the delivery of health care services.

The job requires an introduction, too. To perform this job, what equipment and tools are necessary? What supplies? What type of facilities are used? What about the people who are involved in this job? In addition, the worker, regardless of competence, needs to be introduced to policies, procedures, rules, and regulations if the job is to be performed properly.

Once the worker is oriented, training begins. This may be minimal training for someone coming from a similar job, refresher training to restore certain knowledge and skill to a worker once qualified, or basic job training to a person new to the occupation. Training for promotion and advancement are also part of the total personnel program.

In considering proper and adequate pay, two types of evaluation are necessary. First, the worker's performance should be evaluated in terms of quality, quantity, time, cost and appearance. Second, because certain social and psychological aspects are important to the employment situation, there is a need to evaluate the worker as a person, pointing out what improvements are needed and where the employee excels.

With this type of evaluation, wages can be commensurate with the worth of the performance as well as the worth of the job.

- **There is a need for competent supervisors trained in the practice of human relations.** Unfortunately, one cannot merely select an employee and expect adequate performance to follow automatically. Much greater understanding of the employee and the application of both motivation and incentive are necessary to get good performance. Human relations becomes a necessary tool for achievement of good personnel management.

The many studies of worker wants versus management's understanding of them indicate how little attention has been placed on the intangibles of the employment situation. Too often there is a tendency to concentrate on the wages or benefits or, in other words, the fulfillment of only economic needs.

There is need to begin to understand and know each worker not only as a member of the group but as an individual. What are the employee's needs and how does the employer attempt to satisfy them? What are the employee's values and attitudes? How are they expressed? What is the worker's self-concept and how does this affect the job or serve as a basis for motivation? What different roles are played by this worker, and how can the job contribute to them? This means the supervisor needs to know more than the worker's name, telephone number and address, and perhaps his time card number.

- **Establish superior and well-understood benefit policies.** Personnel policies in terms of benefits are actually a means, not an end or an objective in themselves. Each policy is designed to fulfill some specific purpose.

  Employee benefits are part of a total wage program. Too often this is not understood or appreciated by the employee, and we find that management continues to put out thousands of dollars every pay period in the so-called benefit area, which neither management nor workers recognize as part of the total wage program. An analysis of the costs of providing these benefits would indicate the importance of educating the employees to this fact.

One of the highest priorities that an institution should have is to provide superior employee benefits designed to contribute to the security and sense of well-being for employees and their families. Some of the more common benefits provided in a comprehensive benefit program are as follows:

Benefits Providing Security

Time Paid and Not Worked

Vacations
Authorized holidays

Bereavement
Personal illness

Health Care Benefits

Hospital
Surgical
Medical
Physicians, X-ray, and laboratory
Major Medical
Dental
Eye Care

Income Protection Benefits

Long and/or short-term disability, as applicable

Survivor Security Benefits

Group life
Accidental death and dismemberment

Retirement Benefits

General retirement plan
Other retirement plans, such as TSAs and IRAs

Miscellaneous Benefits

Service awards
Free parking
Employee credit union
Jury duty pay
Shift differential
Employee counseling
Employee health program
Professional liability insurance
Discounts on services/products
Social activities
Education assistance
Legal and financial services
Day-care services
Dependent life insurance

- **Flexible Benefits.** For the past few years, many health care employees have been asking for "flexible benefits." Flexible benefits offer employees a choice of benefits that more closely respond to their needs. Part of the concept of flexible benefits is to allow employees self-determination in their compensation package. But many institutions make the mistake of considering flexible benefits solely because they anticipate favorable employee reaction. Implementing a flexible plan merely to give employees self-determination can be expensive and yet not a solution to an employee relation problem. Institutions should think carefully about potential advantages weighed against the cost, both in work hours and actual cost outlay. Designing a flexible benefit program should be done only after consultation and advice from compensation professionals.

- **Hidden Paychecks.** Many employees see their benefit plans as essentially inactive, getting some good out of them only when triggered by a specific event such as sickness, accident, or death. Personalized annual benefit reports, distributed to individual employees, help transform the inactive perception about benefits. It reveals the benefit program at work on a day-to-day basis and shows how the benefits provide continued security for the employee and family.

  The report should display, in a simple format, present and projected benefit amounts for each event, eligibility requirements, effective dates, and a wide range of benefit-related information. There are a number of qualified consulting firms that will properly design personalized benefit reports for a minimal fee per employee serviced.

- **Effective communication.** As we have emphasized, communication is a vital tool. For health care managers, it is a tool for expressing ideas, making assignments, and evaluating performance. There should be not only a downward flow of communication, but an upward flow as well, and--to eliminate isolationism--horizontal communication within the organization. Communication should be planned as other tools are planned, so that there is a specific objective to be attained. It is important to determine, for example, what should be communicated, when, by whom, and through what method. There needs to be a method of gaining feedback to be sure that the communication reached the right party with a proper interpretation. We cannot assume that each supervisor and department head is equally able to communicate, or that all employees glean the same message from a communication.

- **Learn from evaluation of the personnel program by administration and by the worker.** In the cycle of management functions we begin with planning and end with control or the evaluation of what happened compared with what was intended. Certainly in the personnel management activity of the health care facility, evaluation is an important and vital segment. Too often there is little concern on the part of administration for effectively evaluating what is happening in terms of the personnel program. A few statistics are reported periodically but these may or may not have meaning.

For each specific objective set forth for the personnel program, there is need to design a specific method of evaluation. For example, if safety is one objective, appropriate statistics need to be kept on the incidence and frequency of accidents, the amount of lost time, and direct and indirect costs. If employee health is an objective, then specific information is needed on absences due to illness, findings on preemployment, annual physical examinations, and the nature of illnesses. Labor turnover rates, stability rates, and absentee rates are important in the evaluation of the program. The number and nature of grievances, the causes of resignations, and the sources of effective recruits are additional data for this form of evaluation.

Unfortunately, administration too often ignores the need for personnel program evaluation, whereas the employees are constantly evaluating the personnel program. The number and nature of grievances are really an evaluation of the personnel program.

The exit interview is a management tool that can tap the attitude of the worker at the time of discharge or resignation to find what lies behind the actual resignation or discharge. The interview can determine what the worker liked and disliked about the job--the supervisor, the co-workers, the policy, the duties, the tools. This can be coupled with labor turnover analysis to begin to find not only the direct and final cause, but the contributing factors leading to resignations, discharges, and layoffs.

Suggestion systems often bring in more than suggestions, since they can be tabulated into patterns to find out the areas of greatest concern to the employee. Some so-called ''suggestions'' are really grievances expressed in a different way.

Morale surveys have been used effectively to elicit the evaluation of the personnel program as viewed by the employee.

The selection of this type of information from both workers and administration enables the personnel director and administration to make a realistic evaluation of what is occurring compared to what was intended and to take appropriate steps to redesign the personnel program where necessary.

- **Keep comprehensive personnel records for both the job and the worker.** It has been said that the employee's record dies at the moment the employee is hired. Too often this is true. The typical personnel record as viewed in a health care facility might consist of the application blank, a few sketchy interview notes, notice of a reference verification, and results of a physical examination. This is frequently the only information that justifies sending the applicant to the supervisor for final selection or to see if an employee qualifies for a promotion. What, then, needs to be added?

Let us assume the worker has been employed for six years. If we look into the record we will want to find not just the original information, but facts about responses to supervision, progress as a result of training, social relations within the department and with those in other departments, particular ambitions, areas of greatest weakness as well as greatest strengths, and a review of performance. In other words, the employee's record should be a reflection of the employee. See Exhibit 13-1 on how to standardize personnel records.

One additional phase is necessary. Since personnel management is the proper integration of a job and a worker, we need a record of the job. Facts elicited from the job analysis will serve as a basis for this type of record, giving proper identification of the job, summary of activities, and performance requirements. The important point is the content of the total record as another tool to help the health care facility meet its needs and the needs of it workers.

- **Make sure a competent personnel director is in charge of a centralized personnel program.** Even a 25-bed health care facility will find that its personnel program is important enough to be centralized in the hands of the most capable person to carry it out. We have long since given up the idea of each supervisor and department head keeping books on financial transactions and submitting separate and unrelated reports to the administration for the governing board--recognizing that this phase of total administration is important enough to be concentrated into the hands of someone competent to administer this function--but money alone will not operate the health care facility; people with proper skills and motivation are more important. Personnel administration, then, is at least as important as financial administration and needs at least equal attention by management.

In a small institution, this activity might be combined with other assignments and given to the administrator or business manager or one of the major department heads, but the person assigned to the personnel functions ought to be competent to handle them.

In larger facilities of up to roughly 200 employees, there would certainly be justification for a separate and distinct personnel department and the employment of a competent personnel director. Competence requires more than the ability to get along with people. It also requires detailed knowledge and skill in the specific techniques of comprehensive personnel management.

```
XYZ MEDICAL CARE

SUBJECT:  Standardized Content of Employee Personnel Files
POLICY & PROCEDURE NO.  125-28

                                  Effective Date:  10/6/80
                                  Reviewed Date:   9/2/81
                                  Revised Date:    10/8/82,
                                  _____12/16/83
                                  Reviewed Date:   6/84

DEPARTMENT RESPONSIBLE:  PERSONNEL

AUTHORIZATION:            _____
                                  Vice-President
                                  Personnel & Employee Relations


                          _____
                                  President
```

I. *Purpose*

    To establish and standardize the kind of information that will be kept in individual employee personnel files.

II. *Policy*

    A. Official employee personnel files are maintained by and in the Personnel Department.

    B. The following kinds of information and records will be included in the individual's official personnel file:

- Application for employment and/or resumes
- Written references pertaining to employment
- Evidence of licensure or registration required for position held
- Employee performance evaluations
- Training and education achievement records
- Wage assignments and garnishments
- Records on uniforms, keys, and equipment issued
- Correspondence related to employee's insurance coverages
- Records of salary changes and/or deduction authorizations
- Records of other changes in employment status, i.e., standard hours, transfers, promotions, etc.
- Records of lost time due to accidents
- Records of compensable injuries
- Supervisory recommendations, reprimands, and/or written warning notices

Note: As a general rule, unless the employee so designates, grievance procedure records and subjective information about the employee, other than as stated above, will not be retained in the employee's personnel file.

Exhibit 13-1.

```
III. Responsibility
     The vice president--personnel and employee relations, or his
     designee, shall be responsible for administration of this policy.

IV.  Procedure
     Records and materials may be inserted in the personnel files only by
     members of the personnel department staff as delegated by the vice
     president--personnel and employee relations.

V.   Filing Instructions
     This policy shall be filed in Section 125 of the Policy & Procedures
     Manual.

VI.  Distribution
     This policy is to be distributed facility-wide.
```

Exhibit 13-1, cont.

The still larger health care facilities will find that the personnel director cannot perform all activities alone and will likely need specialists to handle employment, job analysis, wage administration, work simplification, training, and other functions.

The personnel department has the responsibility of staffing the health care facility with qualified, well-adjusted employees. It has the responsibility, within delegated authority, for planning and administering a comprehensive personnel program and is responsible directly to the administrator on all matters involving employee problems and relations. It has the responsibility of recruiting and screening job applications and referring them to the department heads for interview.

Personnel administration is the planning, supervision, direction and coordination of those activities of an organization that contribute to realizing the defined purpose of that organization with a minimum of human effort and friction, with an animating spirit of cooperation, and with proper regard for the genuine well-being of all members of the organization.

To keep it simple, yet to clarify several significant points, it could be stated that the purposes of the personnel department are:

- To coordinate the needs of the institution with those of individual employees in such a way as to provide the community with efficient health care service and to staff the facility with qualified, well-adjusted employees.

- To increase the efficiency and effectiveness of the operating departments that directly or indirectly provide care and comfort for the patients and/or clients.

- To work with the employee to assure his maximum service to the department and employing institution and the maximum use of individual capacities resulting in the greatest possible amount of individual and group satisfaction.

- To manage the institution's human resources capabilities and maintain harmonious employee relations.

- To develop and maintain a modern, comprehensive, centrally administered program of human resources and personnel management functions administered on a daily basis by all members of the supervisory staff.

- To recruit and maintain a competent staff capable of efficiently and effectively executing their job responsibilities.

- To assist both the institution and the employees to achieve goals and objectives through the application of accepted personnel administrative practices.

- To assure that the facility is in compliance with applicable federal and/or state employment practices or standards, as well as with other socioeconomic federal or state legislation.

SCOPE OF THE PERSONNEL DEPARTMENT

- Recruitment of applicants for employment

    Employment specifications
    Employment requisition system
    Development of applicant sources
    Recruitment and retention programs

- Pre-employment screening and placement

    Initial employment applications
    Initial screening interviews
    Referrals to department heads or supervisors for selection
    Verification of applicant references

Scheduling pre-employment physical examinations
Completion of employment processing for selected applicants

- Interview/orientation

  Wage and salary review
  Personnel policies and practices review
  Employee social activities
  Employee benefits programs
  Attendance requirements
  Job hazards and safety strategies

- Centralization of all personnel records/statistics

  Compliance with privacy protection legislation
  Applications
  Interview notes
  References
  Status sheets
  Personnel cards and records
  Termination records

- Employee identification

  Identification cards
  Name pins
  File of employee professional licenses and/or professional
  registrations

- Employee information and communication

  Bulletin boards for required federal/state notices to employees
  Payroll inserts as needed
  Special memos and bulletins for employees
  Articles for hospital publications relative to personnel administration

- Personnel policies and practices

  Development of personnel policies and practices
  Publication of personnel policy handbook
  Publication of job hazards and safety strategy handbook
  Publication and yearly update of personnel and labor relations
  policies

- Transfer and promotion program

    Job posting procedure
    Job enrichment

- Employee counseling

    Career goals for employees
    Referral service
    Exit interviews

- Employee benefit programs

    Health insurance
    Pension plan (in compliance with employee retirement income)
    Security Act of 1974
    Holidays
    Life insurance
    Tax-sheltered annuity program
    Sick leave
    Long- and/or short-term disability program
    Employee health program/policies/procedures
    Terminal benefits
    Unemployment insurance compensation
    Workers' compensation program
    Leaves of absence (paid and unpaid)
    Vacation benefits

- Position analysis program

    Master file of job descriptions
    Job evaluation program
    Job analysis
    Position control

- Performance evaluation

    Performance standards (criteria-based guidelines)
    Performance evaluation program (criteria-based)

- Wage and salary administration program

  Internal equity
  External equity
  Career classification system
  Payroll entry processing
  Payroll exit processing
  Wage scales and wage increase system
  Salary administration processes

- Employee relations

  Educational program
  Grievance procedure
  Departmental meetings
  Suggestion box
  Liaison with legal counsel
  Compliance with Fair Labor Standards Act
  Compliance with National Labor Relations Act

- Statistics for management

  Monthly

  Applicants
  Accessions
  Separations
  Turnover
  Stability
  Labor Force
  Risk Management
  Safety loss control statistics

  Annual

  Summary of *monthly* reports (annual report)
  Summary of grievances filed
  Summary of unemployment benefits paid
  Summary of risk management/loss control program

- Research

  Absence factors (as needed)

Employee surveys
Benefit programs competitiveness
Recruitment sources and techniques
Stability factors
Turnover factors
Wage surveys
Risk management/safety techniques

Institute Proper Personnel Management Controls

As with any other facet of management, the personnel program itself needs to build in certain control devices as a guide for what it is doing and as a measure of what is being done. These controls are more than statistical information accumulated and analyzed. They are specific devices established for the purpose of controlling one or more personnel activities.

For example, there is need for a position control program in order to maintain a proper number and variety of workers to accomplish a given amount of work. This might be set up by itself or combined with a total personnel budget that calculates and anticipates the number of hours required by each position and the worth of each hour's labor converted to payroll dollars. The control here is of the work hours; when adhered to, based on original policy, it can become an effective control device.

There are other control devices perhaps not thought of as such. Specific policies, for example, are a control on individual decision-making. A systematized wage administration program is another control device for establishing minimum rates of pay and increments based on tenure and performance. The job specification likewise is a control on the selection of applicants for pending job vacancies. The performance evaluation is another control device to measure what the worker did in contrast to what was expected in his performance.

Role of Computers in Maintaining Records

We are living in a high technology world. John Naisbitt tells us, "As a society, we have been moving from the old to the new. And we are still in motion. Caught between eras, we experience turbulence. Yet, amid the sometimes painful and uncertain present, the restructuring of America proceeds unrelentingly."[1] Staying competitive in today's health care environment demands the most efficient use of human resources. To be able to manage a workforce effectively, administer wages properly, control the number of positions, monitor job specifications, control attendance, regulate job variances, and administer performance evaluations, the personnel department needs to be automated.

An institution-wide information base capable of flexible response to internal personnel management needs and external regulatory requirements must be health care executives' top priority in the 1980s. The key to effective personnel management and related decision-making in health care institutions is timely, accurate, and reliable information on every aspect of the institution's personnel administration program.

Computerization of personnel information in health care institutions is a necessity. It must be done, it must be done correctly, and the program selection process must involve top management. Effective personnel computer systems require not only dependable hardware and sophisticated software but, even more, planning and self-education on the part of the human resource practitioners.

Human resource management systems are available from a variety of management computer companies. The systems available offer some or all of the components necessary for cost-effective human resource management, such as:

- Payroll-wage data

- Benefit administration

- Safety and health

- Applicant flow

- Position control and position history

- Attendance control

- Applicant tracking

- Flexible compensation

- Staff planning

- Time reporting

- EEO and affirmative action reporting

- Departmental action notices

- Employee profiles

- Labor complement profiles

As more changes take place in the health care industry, those health care institutions that have the information readily on hand to make timely personnel decisions are going to be in a better position than other institutions that are unprepared for the changes.

ENDNOTES

1. John Naisbitt, *Megatrends: Ten New Directions Transforming Our Lives.* (New York: Warren Books), 1982.

CHAPTER 14

Suggested Personnel Policies and Procedures

The American labor relations system is one of the most legislated in the Western world. No major aspect of the employment relationship is free from regulation or guidelines mandated by either federal or state government. The entire field of labor law in the United States is very dynamic, but at the same time the existing structure regulates the actions and decisions of employers with such specificity that experimentation and innovation are greatly inhibited. It is extremely important that personnel policies and procedures be carefully reviewed by legal counsel to ensure that the institution is not inadvertently creating either contractual obligations with its employees or, from an employee relations point of view, causing union activity by employees.

These legal and socioeconomic forces have created sensitive and demanding elements that need to be considered when developing personnel policies and procedures. For this reason it is important not only to clarify the job to be performed and the wages to be received for adequate performance, but also to clarify all other aspects of the employee-employer relationship through an extended and expanded set of personnel policies and procedures.

Greater detail is needed. Employees are challenging institutional practices and policies more and more. The employer needs consistency in presenting answers. It is, therefore, essential that the conditions of the worker relationships be clearly determined and presented in written form. The following is a list, not necessarily in priority order, of what should be considered essential personnel policies and procedures. Each of the following should be written and published as a policy, and each policy should have its purpose, scope, eligibility or coverage requirements, balance of considerations, definitions or terms, and possible exceptions in order to be complete and comprehensive.

- **Department: Human Resources**

    Organizational chart for the Department of Human Resources
    Confidentiality of personnel records and reference requests
    Employment and recruitment policies and procedures
    Termination of employment (voluntary and involuntary)
    Grievance procedure
    Job posting program, promotion program, and transfer policy
    Leaves of absence
    Sick leave
    Holidays

Vacations

Pension plan

Wage/Salary administration policy (pay increases, on-call, differentials, etc.)

Rest periods (coffee breaks and meal periods)

Bereavement absences

Benefit program for salaried employees

Jury duty leaves

Change-of-employment information

Discipline

Acknowledgment and recognition of employees upon their retirement

Employment classification

Service awards

Equal employment opportunity and affirmative action

Licensure/registration--mandatory/voluntary

Job classifications and descriptions

Employee adaptation periods

Work week/work day pay periods

Expense approval for required attendance at lectures, meetings and/or training programs

Payment of wages/salaries to nonexempt employees for attendance at lectures, meetings and/or training programs

Sexual harassment

Standardized content of employee personnel files

Harassment--age, physical, mental, race, color, religion, ancestry or national origin

Insurance programs (life, medical, dental)

Personnel procedure for a deceased employee

Variation from standard work day/work week

Exit interviews

Progressive return to full-time duty after a work injury

Appearance, grooming and identification standards

Reduction-in-force and layoff policy

Seniority--service dates, anniversary dates

Performance standards and performance evaluations

Attendance and tardiness

Supplementary employment (salaried employees)

Safety program

Security program

Work clearance for aliens

Communications program

- **Department: Labor Relations**

  Organizational chart for Labor Relations Department
  Labor relations policy (union and/or nonunion)
  Solicitations, distribution of literature, bulletin boards
  Strike preparation plan
  Membership and participation in professional associations and programs
  Management responsibilities and rights
  Arbitration (in a union facility)
  Bargaining (in a union facility)

- **Department: Education and Management Development**

  Organizational chart for Education and Management Development Office
  Tuition reimbursement program
  Employee orientation program
  Continuing education and staff development
  Scholarship program
  New and/or expanded educational endeavors
  Employee continuing education records
  Guest relations program
  Management development program

- **Department: Employee Health**

  Organizational chart for Employee Health Office
  Pre-employment health evaluations
  Employee yearly health evaluations
  Employee immunizations
  Return to work after illness or work-related injury (for hourly and salaried employees), other than for illnesses
  Confidentiality of employee health records
  Payment for employee health services
  Rubella titers
  Administration of allergy material
  Hepatitis B serology screening of new employees
  Reporting of occupational illnesses/injuries
  Needle puncture wounds
  Chemically dependent employees
  Employee health office involvement/responsibility in nonwork-related illnesses and injuries
  Progressive return to full work duty after a work-related injury

Policy on pregnant employees
Hepatitis B immunization
Caring for patients with or suspected to have acquired immune deficiency syndrome (AIDS)
Smoking policy

POLICY AND PROCEDURE FORMAT

This chapter identifies a popular format used to record and communicate policies and procedures. The styles can vary; however, certain elements should be included in all written policies and procedures. These are:

- Purpose of the policy

- Name of person or department responsible for administering the policy

- Procedure that needs to be followed to put the policy in motion

- A distribution section clearly defining who needs to get the policy and how it will be communicated.

Exhibit 14-1 depicts a policy format, including how the form should be structured and, most importantly, the distribution element.

Exhibit 14-2 depicts, in more detail, what each of the sections should contain in order for the policy to be complete. Specific instructions are written into Exhibit 14-2 to assist in the writing process.

Exhibit 14-3 depicts a completed policy on employee relations for Express Care, Inc., a Division of the XYZ Medical Center.

There are many causes of personnel problems and many sources from which they arise. Each problem may have more than one cause, and this perhaps is one reason personnel problems are often so apparently difficult to solve. Poorly written or nonexistent personnel policies often create problems.

It is evident that the whole American health care delivery system has entered a new era. To maintain the proper balance between employer and employee rights and obligations, policies and procedures are critical. Personnel policies and procedures can be the starting point in maintaining or improving patient care, personnel relations, public relations, and human relations.

Clarifying policies and procedures is good business. By doing so, the institution is forced to define its goals and the strategies employed to reach them. Policies and procedures are also good morale builders because they let employees know for certain what is expected of them. Clearly defined, well-written, and properly communicated personnel policies and procedures are a reflection of the facility's corporate culture.

```
EXPRESS CARE, INC.
A Division of XYZ Medical Center

SUBJECT:_____
POLICY & PROCEDURE NO.  _____

                                  Effective Date:  _____
                                  Revised:    _____-_____
                                  Reviewed:   _____

DEPARTMENT RESPONSIBLE:  _____

AUTHORIZATION:
                                  _____
                                  Department Head(s)
                                  Committee Chairman
                      (or)        Management Team Member
                      (or)        Chief of Staff
                      (or)        President
```

I. *Purpose*

The first section should be a brief statement covering the purpose
of the policy to enable readers to easily ascertain the subject
matter covered. Subsequent paragraphing of all sections should be
identified with alphabetical characters or numbers as appropriate.

   I. (Section)

      A. Major Paragraph

         1. Sub-Paragraph

           a.

              (1)

                 (a)

II. *Policy*

The second section should be a brief policy statement concerning the
subject matter covered.

III. *Responsibility*

The third section should identify the organizational member,
department or service (by title) responsible for various parts of
the procedures with a general statement of scope of responsibility
for accomplishment.

IV. *Procedure*

The fourth section should present the how, when, what, and where of
the procedure designed to carry out the policy as stated in Section
II. This section and subsequent numbered paragraphs will constitute
the bulk of most statements.

V. *Distribution*

The section should delineate the appropriate departments to receive
the policy.

VI. *Filing Instructions*

The final section should provide reference to any previously filed
policy and describe the action to be taken in respect to the old
policy and filing of the new one. Also, someone needs to consider
to what degree the policy provisions need to be communicated and to
whom.

Exhibit 14-1.

EXPRESS CARE, INC.
A Division of XYZ Medical Center

SUBJECT: (short title or subject)
POLICY & PROCEDURE NO. _____

Effective Date: _____
Revised Dates: _____

Reviewed Dates: _____

DEPARTMENT RESPONSIBLE: _____

AUTHORIZATION: _____

(Note: This model should be used throughout the institution)

I. *Purpose*

This statement should establish the policy, procedures, and responsibilities concerning the issuance of official publications covering directive and informational material for use within the institution.

Definition: A **policy** shall be defined as an authoritative, written statement of fact that serves to embody the philosophy of and lend direction to the establishment and accomplishment of the accountability objectives of the organization.

II. *Policy*

A. Policy statements should be initiated by the responsible committee, department head/management team member, approved by the responsible management team representative, and authenticated by any or all of the following, as appropriate: committee chairperson, responsible department head(s), management team representative(s), chief of staff, or President. All departments within the institution should write and issue policies in the same style and format.

B. All policy statements so issued should be reviewed annually, revised (if appropriate), and reissued with the date of review or revision affixed. The date of original issue should always be recorded on each policy. Original policies and copies of all revisions should be kept indefinitely in a master file.

III. *Responsibility*

General responsibility should be delegated as indicated in the following:

A. Management team--Assurance that all policies and procedures within its area of control are up-to-date, reflect current modes of operation, are reviewed by appropriate individuals/ departments, and comply with current standards of practice (e.g., accreditation standards, state licensing standards, Fair Labor Standards Act, National Labor Relations Act.) It is highly advisable that personnel and labor relations policies and

Exhibit 14-2.

procedures be reviewed by legal counsel before finalization and distribution.

B. Administration office--Coordination, publication, and distribution of all policies; maintenance of a master file set; and assurance of annual review. Publication of an index of policies alphabetically by department and by numerical index.

C. Department heads--Initiation, preparation, review, revision, and authentication, as appropriate. Maintenance of a file set of departmental policies, pertinent interdepartmental policies, and hospital-wide policies; and assurance that appropriate information is disseminated to all employees within the department.

D. All employees--Read or be familiar with publications, as appropriate, and abide by the policies set forth.

IV. *Procedure*

(Should present the how, what, when, and where)

A. Policy Formulation--Policies that affect the entire organization should be promulgated and implemented by administration. All other policies will be the responsibility of the department head most affected or having the greatest responsibility for implementation, as discerned by the department head or administration.

Policies should be submitted in draft form to the department head's management team member. The management team member may approve, refer to higher authority, and/or refer the proposed policy back to the department head for coordination with other departments for revision, as necessary.

After these actions have been taken and final review carried out, the originating person or department is responsible for preparation of the final policy statement for necessary authentication and distribution.

B. Policy review--The responsible administrative official or department head should review at the time of initiation, and annually thereafter on the anniversary date of each policy, all policies that are within his area of responsibility. This review should consist of at least the following:

1. Applicability--Is the policy still necessary?

2. Currency--Is the policy current and up-to-date in all respects?

3. Coordination--Is the administrative official/department head aware of any requirements of his policy that may conflict with the policies of another department? If so, necessary coordinating actions shall be taken and the policy modified as necessary and resubmitted for approval and authentication. Has the policy been distributed to those areas/departments involved?

4. Any policy that may have an impact upon or be of concern to the medical staff should be forwarded to the president or, in his absence, the vice-president--operations for review and consideration by the medical staff (if deemed appropriate).

Exhibit 14-2, cont.

5. Any policy that may have financial implications should be reviewed with the vice-president--finance prior to finalization.

6. Any policy that may have an impact upon personnel matters should be reviewed with the vice-president--personnel prior to final approval.

7. Any policy proposed by a medical staff committee should be reviewed with the executive committee of the medical staff and the appropriate member(s) of the management team prior to finalization and implementation. The administration office should be responsible for sending out notification of an annual comprehensive review of each department's policies. Administration and department heads should report results of their review in writing within 30 days to their immediate superior. These reports should be filed in the administration office.

V. *Distribution*

Policies should be distributed hospital-wide to all departments that can be affected by the policy provisions.

VI. *Filing Instructions*

This section should contain instructions relative to actions to be taken with respect to the previous policy and the filing of the new one. For example, does the policy need to be communicated before it is filed?

Exhibit 14-2, cont.

```
EXPRESS CARE, INC.
A Division of XYZ Medical Center

SUBJECT:  Employee Relation Policy
POLICY & PROCEDURE NO.  90-1

                                    Effective Date:  10/20/75
                                    Reviewed:  2/3/81, 2/4/82,
                                               2/22/83, 6/4/85
                                    Revised:  _____

DEPARTMENT RESPONSIBLE:             _____
                                    Vice-President--Personnel and
                                    Employee Relations

AUTHORIZATION:                      _____
                                    President
```

I. *Purpose*

The board of directors of the XYZ Medical Center has set forth the basic employee relations policy of the institution in a Statement of Policy adopted on October 20, 1975.

We believe that voluntary commitment to these policies, our adherence to them through effective management, and good supervision and direct communication with our employees, are the best ways to maintain fair, constructive relations with all employees at Express Care, Inc.

II. *Policy*

As attached.

III. *Responsibility*

The effective administration of this policy necessitates commitment and involvement of everyone in a management or supervisory capacity. The vice-president--personnel and employee relations will be responsible for administering and monitoring those areas listed in the Statement of Policy. Department heads and supervisors will be responsible for those aspects related to working conditions, fair and adequate supervision, opportunity for employees to express themselves in policy matters, interest in employees' personal problems and encouraging use of the grievance procedure. The administration of Express Care, Inc. will be responsible for coordinating, publicizing, and enforcement of the policy and its provisions.

IV. *Procedure*

Department heads and supervisors must be constantly receptive and responsive to the labor relations climate in their respective areas and immediately discuss with the vice-president--personnel and employee relations any perceived problems.

V. *Filing Instructions*

This policy shall be filed in Section 90 of the Policy and Procedures Manual.

VI. *Distribution*

This policy must be distributed to all departments and communicated by department heads and supervisors to all employees of Express Care, Inc.

Exhibit 14-3.

XYZ MEDICAL CENTER   October 20, 1975

STATEMENT OF POLICY

EMPLOYEE RELATIONS POLICY

The XYZ Medical Center believes in, is practicing, and will continue to practice fair employee relations policies.

The XYZ Medical Center is dedicated to promoting an atmosphere of wholesome cooperation among all of its employees that they may realize the maximum satisfaction and personal fulfillment from their work. We are pledged to do all that is reasonably possible to meet the needs of our total staff and to foster and promulgate the following for all regardless of occupation, profession, race, religion, sex, age, creed, color, national origin, or handicap.

- Competitive wage and salary programs
- Competitive benefit programs
- Desirable working conditions
- Fair and adequate supervision
- Fair promotion and transfer programs
- Steady employment
- Adequate financial security at retirement
- Opportunity to express oneself in policy matters
- Progressive personnel programs
- Educational programs for career mobility
- Occupational safety and health standards
- Interest in employees' personal problems
- Equal employment programs
- Grievance procedure

Because of these, we believe that unions (or quasi-unions) are not necessary to protect the best interests of our employees or those of our patients. Where there is a formal progressive personnel administration program designed to create conditions under which employees can be fairly compensated, with socioeconomic opportunities, good working conditions, good supervision and an opportunity for growth, there is no need for third parties and third party tactics to intervene between our employees and the management of the XYZ Medical Center.

We believe that our voluntary adherence to these principles is the best policy for our employees and that their interests are best served by our direct voluntary action in their behalf and by their direct personal communication with us. We believe there is no need for a union at the XYZ Medical Center in order to obtain these ends.

As a good corporate citizen, we will comply with the applicable laws and regulations in respect to labor unions and will act in good faith with any union certified as the representative of our employees. We hope, however, that the majority of our employees are of the conviction,

Exhibit 14-3, cont.

as we are, that it is better to continue to discuss with us directly any concern they may have.

We believe further that we should make our views known to all employees, if necessary, and should discuss frankly the disadvantages to all concerned if a union attempts to intervene in the XYZ Medical Center.

We pledge ourselves to do all we can to continually further the interests of our employees and to continually assure equitable pay and working conditions for all employees at the XYZ Medical Center.

The preceding Statement was approved by the XYZ Medical Center Board of Trustees on October 20, 1975, and is so reflected in the minutes of that meeting.

Exhibit 14-3, cont.

CHAPTER 15

Corporate Culture: Maintaining the Voluntary Approach

Corporate culture reflects a company's or a health care institution's breeding and evolution. It includes the operational situations, conditions, inner customs, rituals, values, and just "the way things are done around here." Corporate culture influences many day-to-day activities, and impacts heavily upon not only the future of the institution, but also the employee-management relations. There is a growing awareness of the importance of corporate culture to all health care institutions, particularly as they cope with multiple changing environments brought about by new reimbursement systems and new methodologies in the delivery of health care. Health care facilities are labor intensive, and since employees are so closely involved in an institution's culture, it behooves management to periodically evaluate its operational situations to determine where it stands relative to corporate culture.

As operational conditions are reviewed, it is important to be mindful that there is often a strong sense of unity among the employees. These are first one's peers, associates, or co-workers, who often share one's commonality of interests, achievements or frustrations. At times employees believe they and management are in two camps-the "we" and "they"--rather than in distinct but collaborative roles. In more severe conditions there is often the feeling that employees need protection from management.

Obviously these are all conditions that suggest the relationship between the employee and management is poor and the real sense of team effort has not yet been achieved. It must be recognized that the condition, even if it does not affect a particular employee directly but instead affects a co-worker, may in fact have a ripple effect throughout the total group of employees, who tend to put themselves in the shoes of the affected worker and thus secure the feelings of that worker as though it were personal. The fallout from this practice is negative morale.

The following conditions are, therefore, identified for reflective review as a management checkup on its corporate culture:

1. *Discharge,* the punishment that separates an employee from his means of earning a living, is obviously the ultimate destroyer of any relationship. The very act ceases the relationship, and only legal implications of rights and benefits might sustain some lingering shadow of the relationship that has already ceased to be. To what extent have employees viewed discharges as malicious, capricious, or arbitrary? In the interest of protecting the rights of the affected employee, has management avoided presenting a balanced view of the situation, leaving other employees to

judge management's behavior based solely on the one-sided position of the discharged worker? What is management's justification for this action? Has there been adequate warning--verbal and written--and does the record document such efforts?

2. The *layoff* is a temporary separation of the employee from the job and is enforced upon hospitals and nursing homes through the necessity of cost containment programs by which actual costs of operations are related to income from such operations. Because the health care facility has a fluctuating census, it needs means to increase staffing with high census and adjust downward staffing under conditions of low census. Layoff in itself creates major problems of insecurity. It also questions the appropriate use of seniority versus the possible use of merit. How has the facility handled part-time, short-time or indefinite layoffs. To what extent has seniority or merit been recognized and accepted from the employee point of view?

3. *Wages* and the further aggravation of wage rates by inadequate recognition of rate adjustments or performance improvement merit adjustments create much frustration to health care personnel. Health care personnel feel a marked sense of injustice when the daughter of the weekend nurse can earn as much as her parent by working as a supermarket clerk. Employees who have made an effort to improve their qualifications and increase productivity feel deprived in reaction to a meager response to what they view as a major effort. To what extent are these real situations in the facility?

4. *Inconsistent interpretation and enforcement* of personnel policies, practices, rules and regulations can leave an employee uncertain, confused, resentful, frustrated and sometimes desiring to challenge such conditions to make them right. Whether intended or not, unequal treatment under similar conditions will be viewed as partiality and perhaps as open discrimination. Are supervisors instructed on the intent, content, and appropriate interpretations of policies, practices and rules? Do they have definitions of terms, written procedures, and other aids to assure consistency in both interpretation and enforcement?

5. To be confronted daily by an *inadequate supervisor* subjects an employee to an ongoing relationship that is continually unsatisfactory. Employees resent the supervisor who is unstable, displays temper, becomes emotional, fails to listen, is noncommunicative, does not seek advice, does not follow through on recommendations, and/or does not report back on the status of conditions. There is further objection to the supervisor who practices nepotism, enjoys favoritism, fails to give appropriate

recognition to the identity of employees, denies respect, and/or fails to involve the employee as a partner in decision-making, problem-solving dialogue. The employee is further critical of the supervisor who may personally lack competency, does not enjoy support of higher management, displays inconsistent behavior, lacks self-assurance, uses employees' ideas as their own, and may require ego satisfaction at the expense of the employee. To what extent do these factors describe any of the supervisors, department directors or administrative personnel?

6. The basic belief by employees that there is no effective means by which to settle or resolve *grievances*--despite the existence of grievance systems, grievance policies, or even grievance committees--looms as a major sign of "no confidence." The fear of resentment even if there were to be no reprisal may be sufficiently strong to place the grievance system in a formidable position. Belief that a grievance filed through the grievance system would not receive objective and fair settlement would further deter use of the system. Employees question whether management can truly be objective about grievances. They also worry that management keep records of grievances and their solutions and that an employee using the grievance system will some day live to regret it.

   To what extent do these conditions prevail? How often has the grievance system been used, and did it support management or the employee? What did the employee think? Did management again lose employee understanding by attempting to protect the rights of privacy while the grieving employee publicized the grievance conditions throughout the workforce?

7. The *lack of effective two-way communication* often prevents establishing any type of relationship. Employees not only want to be kept informed by higher levels of management within the organization, thus increasing the credibility of the communication itself, but also want to know that upward communication is equally possible--to immediate supervisors, department directors or even top administration. There may be a system that provides communication too late, so that it follows the grapevine. The information may be too little to meet the need to feel informed. It may concern topics that interest management but do not yet interest the employee. The communication pipeline requires not only that the employees' eyes and ears be open to what is written or said by higher management but also that management's eyes and ears be tuned to what is being communicated by the employee. Communication requires as its basic condition that there be two involved and interested employees. To what extent do these conditions prevail?

8. The *lack of a sense of a future*--being limited in personal growth, job advancement, career promotion or economic improvement--suggests the absence of a true career system that is organized and is available to employees. The failure to post jobs as a means of notifying employees of possible opportunities; the lack of attention to staff development, in-service training, or continuing education that would lead to the qualifications that would make advancement and promotion possible--all these suggest that an employee's future must be determined solely by his own effort and that no one truly cares.

By providing for approved continuing education units within the hospital, tuition reimbursement plans, attendance at in-service training and continuing education programs, management becomes a party to providing for a future--and, given today's rapidly changing work situation, possibly the "present."

Are employees aware of those who are advanced or promoted and what their investment had to be to qualify? Does each employee have a career destiny as a long-range plan, with short-range goals to assure eventual achievement? Exactly what is the future that is available to a short-term employee who wants to become a long-time health career worker?

9. The *incompetent employee*--one who lacks appropriate knowledge or skill or who has been inappropriately oriented or inadequately trained--becomes a burden to fellow workers. Often an older worker is assigned as a "buddy" to the new worker to assure that the newcomer adjusts smoothly to the organization, the work environment, and the job. This often results in an attachment of the dependent employee on the more productive employee, which aggravates an already established burden.

It is the responsibility of management to recruit appropriately qualified candidates, screen them for assurance of qualifications, and select those who can be productive. Management must introduce the employee to the environment; provide for initial training to show how to apply basic competency factors to the work, procedures, and methods established; and initiate the continuing education by which such an employee maintains his competency. Do these practices prevail as routine?

10. *Automation* and labor saving devices--computers, vertical and horizontal material movers, electronic observation devices, and other such cost-saving and quality improvement conditions--often results in a great sense of fear or insecurity about one's job, and thus resentment and open resistance. There is need to involve the employees in the continuing process of recommending improvements, so that progress is made through the proposals of personnel creating commitments to change rather than inviting resistance to change by imposition of new and different means of getting the job done. Are employees involved? Do they have a voice

in proposing change? Is change made only after the notification of change with supportive reasons and the opportunity for reaction, criticism and alternate proposals?

11. The lack of *discipline* or the inappropriate use of discipline can often disturb the relationship of the employee with management, particularly when employees want to express pride in their work and in the institution. Discipline is mere adherence to standards. Since this might be expected of all, then the failure to exercise discipline is often viewed as a form of favoritism or unequal treatment. It reflects an inconsistency in management's expectations from employees. It creates an instability in the relationship since one is never certain whether to expect discipline when needed or not. Is there an appropriate disciplinary policy with meaningful procedures that is understood by supervisors, practiced as needed, and documented for purposes of review and justification of such actions?

12. The overly demanding, critical, accusative, nonsupportive professional or technical specialist (whether it be a doctor, nurse, or paraprofessional) often creates a sense of disillusionment and disgust among less highly trained employees who would under different circumstances look up to such individuals and show respect. To what extent do such situations exist as routines, as periodic outbursts, or as individual behavior patterns and how do they affect employees? What groups of employees are affected by this behavior?

   Professionals and paraprofessionals must recognize that the dignity of the person is not related to the work that person performs. The need for balanced respect for one another is essential in any effort to build a team.

13. Professionalism no longer stands alone as the primary interest in *safeguarding the care of the patient* and being mindful of the quality of the care that must be delivered. The significance of the facility is made real when the linen handler, the dishwasher, the floor cleaner can join ranks with the therapist, the technologist, the nurse, or the physician in contributing through their own means and efforts to the quality care of the patient. Incompetent, inconsistent, or negligent patient care not only violates the idealism that often adds dignity to the most lowly job but also may overshadow the job objectives that justify concerned effort. Are there means of assuring quality care for patients? Are employees made aware of standards, audits, and results? Are employees involved in the critiques aimed at producing improvement?

14. The establishment of unrealistic or *unattainable performance standards* may often create a sense of pressure or frustration or even create a sense

of inferiority when one cannot attain what may be expected. We suggest that performance standards be established at 110 percent of what an average worker would normally do, thereby requiring some reach or effort for achievement. Once the average worker can achieve the standards, it is time to review them and revise them upward through input and cooperation of affected personnel. Unknown performance standards do not serve to motivate or to set goals for achievement. They may in fact create an atmosphere of instability and uncertainty.

15. *Obsolete* operational practices, policies, procedures, methods, equipment, and supplies may all cluster as a major sign of deterioration that contrasts sharply to the inherent desire to be progressive and to update the operation. An atmosphere of obsolescence can diminish one's pride and in time even one's self-respect. It reflects an atmosphere of losers, not winners. To what extent is there aggressive management behavior to update jobs, procedures, and methods; to revise policies; to replace equipment; to modernize supplies, etc.? Do the employees see the consequences of these efforts?

16. *Unfair performance appraisals* that tend to be based on personalities rather than performance patterns, that tend to be based on indirect or secondhand rather than direct or firsthand information, that tend to be done by a remote rather than an immediate supervisor, that tend to be critical rather than constructive, all result in frustration. Employees may feel they have no means of knowing whether management is aware of efforts to improve performance and will in time reward such effort. The good employee wants his or her performance evaluated and wants the assurance that positive effort is first recognized and will then be rewarded. Does the present performance appraisal system truly evaluate performance, or is it based on personality traits and human virtues? It is objective and constructive, and does it relate to reward?

17. *Wasted resources*--whether unwise expenditures or underutilized facilities and equipment, abused supplies and materials, or even incompetent coworkers--result in serious concerns in the minds of the employees since the resulting waste is reflected in money that could have been added to wages, benefits, or improvements in patient care. The greater the degree of exposure to waste, the greater the degree of diminished confidence in the decisions of management. Where, of recent date, might employees view management's decisions as wasteful? Can management offset the employees' continuing blame of management by attempting to involve the employees in balanced participation in the control of waste?

18. Whether true or not, the beliefs among employees that *morale* is low, that there is too much griping and complaining, that there is backstabbing and personalized gossip, that labor turnover is excessive, and that good personnel do not want to work in the present environment, will make employees behave as though the morale is bad. Where these conditions exist, there is the probability that a morale problem exists. How is morale measured? Does management have a means to detect an increase in such problems? Can management give voice to the employees to participate in means of reducing employee tension and improving morale?

19. *Changes* made too fast and/or too frequently with inadequate advance notice can create an unstable environment and put employees under stress. The extent to which a supervisor seeks advice or recommendations on change and permits an opportunity for the employee to contribute ideas that will lead to improvements often minimizes the resistance to change while diminishing the communication problem that relates to it. Is there this type of participative involvement by employees? Progress requires that changes be made in jobs, personnel, policies, systems, procedures, methods, and techniques. Cooperation requires that employees be party to the process, not its victims.

20. The image or the *reputation of the institution* as an employer or as a provider of health care often becomes essential to the development and maintenance of a sense of pride and a sense of self-respect for being a party to the operation. Conditions that tend to enhance the facility's image in the community create pride and appreciation. Conditions that result in deterioration of that image or reputation initiate problems. What is the image of the institution in the community as an employer, or as a provider of health care services, or as an institution of significance? Is there a difference in the image of the institution among past patients in contrast to present patients? Among active physicians in contrast to the inactive physicians? Or in the minds of civic and business leaders compared to John Q. Public?

21. *Poor security benefits* often stimulate other problems of security, confidence, and relations. It is important, therefore, that employees understand what the employer does provide as a means of enhancing the employee's sense of security. Although there is the need to avoid paternalism, employees still want to know that their families would be protected upon their death, that they have continuous income if they must attend funerals, that retirement is both possible and probable when they reach older age, that there is income protection if one is sick, that health care costs are covered through hospitalization and medical forms of insurance, and that special needs are cared for (such as the job descriptions

to know one's job, the wage systems to know one's compensation, the policy books to know one's work environment, and supervisory conferences to maintain one's relationships.)

22. The adequacy of the *staffing pattern* versus the workload often becomes a major factor in employee insecurity. Excessive workload; working alone, shorthanded, or without relief; uncertainty of working on callback or being pulled, floated, reassigned, doubled over or doubled back--all raise serious concern in the mind of the employee with regard to the adequacy of staffing. It is important to understand that staffing is not just having an available body. There must be adequate competency from available staff, the staff must be assigned the appropriate work for their levels of competency, the work must be designed with appropriate procedures and methods, and the workers must have sufficient motivation that the available staff is as efficient and effective as possible. Do these conditions exist?

23. There may be *factors outside the facility* that contribute to employee-management relations problems, such as high unemployment rates that stimulate a sense of insecurity, excessive government controls that reflect waste and frustration, or unfair legislation that handicap performance or inhibit growth. Health care facilities can no longer exist in a vacuum, and there is need to be alert to the impact the community has on the facility as well as the impact the facility has on the community.

It might seem that there is no end to the list of concerns that could disrupt the effective relationship of employees with management. Each of the foregoing conditions could be expanded and could have many additional implications. Although different groups of employees may express somewhat different patterns of priority, the list to a considerable extent reflects the sequence of importance in such factors. However, there are other conditions that may contribute to the problems initiated by the above points and that need to be reviewed as still further areas for a management checkup. These include:

- Perpetuation of periodic displays of *authoritarianism* and autocratic leadership in contrast to the expected more democratic or participatory styles of management relations. The concept of theory X versus theory Y is generally understood at the employee level today.[1] The employee knows that the response is best when there is a more democratic style of leadership. Management needs a constant reminder that in a democracy one manages at the pleasure of the managed. By united effort the authority of management can be turned off operationally.

- *Poor, wrong or no information* at the time of employment can contribute largely to an initial sense of insecurity that may persist long after the need for insecurity is gone. To what extent are employees satisfied by their initial contacts with the facility in their first ventures through orientation to the hospital, department, and job?

- The *lack of use of seniority* often diminishes in the mind of the employee the sense that there is value in continued loyalty in remaining on the job. The worker wants to build a stake in the job, and to the extent that it cannot be done through recognized merit, it must be done through identified seniority. Is seniority recognized in policies and practices?

- *Inadequate availability of necessary resources* to perform the job--tools and apparatus, supplies and materials, co-workers--results in both insecurity and a lack of confidence in management's ability to manage. The work itself should specify the nature of the resources required for performance, even including the qualifications of the incumbent worker. To what extent is work under this type of descriptive control and is it used in such matters?

- Disbelief or *little hope that administration will act,* communicate, or take corrective action to resolve problems often emerges as the major deficiency in employee confidence in management. Announced actions with target dates and with timely and effective communication to show appropriate execution are important means of establishing credibility. Do these exist? Do the employees accept what is presented? Are the problems that management thinks it has solved in fact solved at the employee level?

- When the *personnel department is viewed as the pawn* of administration and the personnel program is viewed as a management program, there is a loss of any internal mechanism through which the employees feel represented and supported other than the strength of the relationships with the immediate supervisor. The employee is the business of the personnel director and the personnel office. The personnel program must be designed to meet the needs of the employees as the employees meet the needs of the institution. Is there assurance that the personnel office fulfills this vital function and that the personnel director has the respect of the workforce as a resource that they can utilize?

- *Work assignments that are not in job descriptions* add to insecurity and suggest that employees have no protection from being accused of failure in performance when they may not have been aware that performance was expected. Employees tend today to lean heavily on job descriptions as sources of protection, but the job descriptions must be updated, complete, and accurate, as well as adhered to.

- When employees feel that their *supervisors are either unavailable or not responsive,* there is a tendency to become dependent on the co-worker for orientation, training, assistance, and support in grievance settlement. Employees resent a sense of dependency but, although we seek independence, the reality is a true recognition that we are each interdependent with one another. The dependency on co-workers often reflects a deficiency of the supervisors in the mind of the employees.

- *Inappropriate work assignments,* such as work not evenly distributed, not appropriately assigned based on competency of the performer, or inconsistent with the content of the job description, all tend to create insecurity and resentment that undermine confidence in management. Employees seek a sense of fairness and balance in the working situation. To what extent is work properly and fairly assigned?

- The *lack of expressed appreciation,* praise, or individual recognition suggests that no one cares and there is no reward for the effort expended. When the only reward is the paycheck, other problems emerge. Do employees feel appreciated and is praise as readily given as criticism?

- *Working either above or below one's level of competency* can create insecurity or frustration or both. In time, consistent inappropriate work assignments undermine confidence in management. Do the supervisors understand the competency level of employees, and have these been compared with the performance requirement levels of the work?

- *Too may bosses* not only create confusion but also undermine confidence and destroy security. Each worker should have one boss. Although there is an ultimate authority over the worker, there must still be an identifiable proximate authority. This requires appropriate review of the organizational structure and relationships.

- *Discord* among members of the board of trustees; between the board and the administrative staff; within the administrative staff; among the board, the administrative staff, and the medical staff; or among the members of the medical staff--all lead to potential dangers of employee unrest. When the top of the structure shakes, the bottom of the structure will also. In time, the employees will believe there is cause for concern, and this leads to insecurity. Is there harmony in the top echelons of board, administration and medical staff?

- *Interpersonal conflict among employees* can become an important problem for management to resolve. Tension or friction between professionals and subprofessionals, between subprofessionals and nonprofessionals, between the medical areas and the service areas, between the shifts, between departments--all tend to challenge the organization and its strength.

- The *lack of inter- and intra-departmental cooperation* and the lack of interpersonal cooperation suggests that each must do his own with or without the support of others. Cooperation is a beginning point for team effort. It recognizes that each one is important in the organization and that all contribute to the ultimate purpose of the facility. Is there a cooperative spirit that is self-evident in observing the employee at work?

A collective review of these considerations at the management level should identify other peripheral issues. The impact of these thoughts on the present status of the employee-management relationship should be viewed as a starting point in improving an institution's corporate culture. Having a healthy culture will assist both management and employees to cope with the environmental changes in the American health care system.

Management and employees can work together as participating partners in providing the best health care available and can derive mutual satisfaction from their employment. In the words of two experts in human resources, "A climate must be created in which one of two things occur: the individuals in the organization either perceive their goals as being the same as the goals of the organization; or, although different, see their goals as being satisfied as a direct result of working towards the goal of the organization."2

ENDNOTES

1. Douglas McGregor incorporated the perceptions of the capabilities of people in his formulation of Theory X and Theory Y. In essence, Theory X represents a series of personal beliefs held by managerial personnel about people who work for them, namely that people generally prefer to be told what to do and not to think for themselves. Theory Y represents a more positive view, namely that people are capable of setting goals for themselves, and with the right combination of reinforcement and rewards will pursue them vigorously.

2. Bart Metzger and Norman Metzger, "Human Resource Managers Must Provide Democratic Leadership," *Human Resources Newsletter* (July/August 1984: 1-2).

CHAPTER 16

The Role of Participative Management in Employee Relations

A major factor in ensuring good employer-employee relations is participative management. Participative management is more than a written program of how to get along through working together. It is a philosophy that must be carried out in earnest by everyone in the organization. Participative management cannot succeed if only a few individuals actually believe in it and others only pay lip service to the idea. To be successful, participants must have management's confidence in the potentialities of their subordinates, management's awareness of their dependence on the subordinates for a smooth-running organization, and an acceptance of the possible negative consequences of too much emphasis on strict managerial authority.

Less than 100 years ago, factory workers had to toil long hours at work that was meaningless to them. The health and safety of the workers was of practically no concern to the employer, since it was much easier to replace the worker than to correct the unsatisfactory conditions that existed. Thus workers were not able to gain satisfaction from their jobs. They were not able to be creative as in the past, when they had taken products through from start to finish. Instead, they often saw only one small process in the production of a product, and maybe never fully understood their role in the total process. With no satisfaction on the job, employees were left with little ambition or pride in their tasks. Therefore, they often did just enough to get by and produced only what they had to do to hold their jobs.

Under such conditions, it is not surprising that owners and managers developed certain assumptions about workers; they began to see people as inherently lazy and shirking responsibility. It became necessary, therefore, to force workers to follow strict rules and give them no say in their jobs. They were considered expendable resources whose value was measured only by the amount of goods they were able to produce.

Although this attitude that people are lazy and opposed to work is still seen in some of the strict factory systems where workers toil under poor conditions, the rising level of prosperity has significantly improved overall conditions. The high levels of production brought about by technological innovation have enabled people to live better for fewer hours of labor. Because of this increased independence, workers have sought and obtained more say in the work they do. In the society we live in today, it is unacceptable to the majority that a person be forced to work under miserable conditions to obtain the necessities of life.

The traditional theory that people will avoid work whenever possible is no longer accepted by modern management theorists. Research has shown that people truly have a desire to work. It has been found that work is an essential part of a person's life. Work gives a person status and binds him or her to society by providing social acceptability, for work is a social activity. People fear unemployment more than employment since it cuts them off from their social relationships.

The theory of the worker has thus been completely reversed. It is now realized that people will direct and control themselves in achieving goals to which they are committed. Of great importance is the realization that most people seek responsibility and have the capacity to handle complex tasks if given the opportunity and the necessary training. The earlier factory system techniques were not the result of laziness; rather, apparent laziness was the result of the system.

As previously mentioned, people are social beings. They need the acceptance of their peers and neighbors. On the job, they want to feel they are making a contribution, and they want social acceptance and self-esteem. They are concerned with more than monetary awards, and they must be given the chance to prove their worth to the organization and to themselves. This is done through increased emphasis on participative management.

Employees do not need to have a say in all management decisions. This would be impossible. They should, however, be given a say in conditions that directly affect them. The test should be, "Why can't the employee(s) make this decision?" If there is no compelling reason, then the worker(s) should be allowed to decide how a task can best be accomplished. Although management often counters with the argument that the employees will demand more and more decision-making powers and will erode management's authority, this has not been found to be the case. On the contrary, employees are more able to accept the decisions of management when they feel that they are being treated fairly and are being consulted when there are several alternatives available.

Even when it is felt that a decision must be made by management, employees can be informed of the decision and the reasons for it. By being given the opportunity to ask questions and to understand the reasons for a particular decision, they will be better able to accept the decision and will feel more a part of the organization by having been recognized as an integral part of it.

Through participation, employees gain greater control and greater freedom of choice. The opportunity to exert some influence over their own work situation can be repaid to management by loyalty and respect. Management has often found that employees can be invaluable in solving problems that may be much more obvious to them than to the manager who only has a superficial knowledge of the actual situation.

Participation offers substantial opportunities for ego satisfaction for subordinates and can affect their motivation toward obtaining the organizational objectives. Participation can help subordinates feel an integral part of the organization and help them desire to fulfill their obligations faithfully.

Again we emphasize that open, effective communication is the lifeblood of any organization. Without the ability to voice new ideas, to resolve problems, and to remain up-to-date on what is happening, employees cannot do the best possible job or be fully productive. Management must therefore be committed to open, two-way communication for all employees.

There should be at least ten formal communication methods through which concerns, issues, ideas, questions, and grievances can be shared and acted upon. These methods are:

1. *Person to person.* Supervisors have the primary responsibility for maintaining good employee relations; therefore, the first step in any communications process should be employees discussing their issues with their immediate supervisors.

2. *Action needed now.* This is a method by which employees may express opinions, feelings, suggestions, or criticisms and receive a direct response in writing from their immediate supervisor or department head within 72 hours of submitting an Action Needed Now form (see Exhibit 16-1). The completed form may be signed or not, as the employee chooses. If the form is not signed, the response is posted on the departmental bulletin board.

3. *Department meetings.* There should be an opportunity for employees to meet at least once monthly with their department heads for the purpose of becoming informed of what is happening throughout the institution and department. Also, staff members should present issues and concerns to the group for discussion and resolution.

4. *Shift meetings.* Bimonthly shift meetings should be held for the evening and night employees. These meetings afford employees an opportunity to discuss problems they may be experiencing on the off-hour tours of duty. Meetings should be open to all 3-11 and 11-7 employees.

5. *Quality circles.* These are small groups of people who do similar work and meet on a regular basis during work time to identify and solve problems related to the work they perform. Quality circles recommend changes to management and where possible actually implement the changes themselves. Quality circles give the institution the benefit of a vast resource for creative problem solving--the employees closest to the work. Participation in quality circles gives employees the opportunity to express their ideas, effectively communicate with co-workers and other members of the organization, and have a positive impact on the work environment.

XYZ HOSPITAL

ACTION NEEDED NOW

...a program designed to provide a **quick response**
to your questions or areas of concern.

AN AREA OF CONCERN is any situation you are not happy with, a change you would like to see occur, a system that is not working the way you think it should, a situation in which you feel you have not been treated fairly, or anything that is bothering you that you would like to get off your chest.

WITHIN 72 HOURS you will receive a personal written response from your Dept. Head. If you choose not to sign the form, your question and the response will be typed and posted on your department's bulletin board.

Department _____ DATE _____

Area of Concern/Problem:

Suggested Solution: (This section is optional. If you have an idea, here's a chance for you to express it.)

Employee's Name (OPTIONAL!) _____

Action Taken:

Date _____ Dept. Head/Supervisor _____

Exhibit 16-1.

6. *Grievance procedure.* This is the most formal procedure for resolving employee dissatisfactions, issues, or concerns. The first step should be to call for a discussion of the situation with the immediate supervisor. If the problem is not resolvable at this level, the employee should next discuss the situation with his or her department head, at which time a resolution can often be reached. If the grievance is not satisfactorily resolved by the immediate supervisor or department head, the employee should be referred to the vice-president--personnel and employee relations. If, through conference, satisfaction or settlement of the grievance cannot be obtained, the vice-president--personnel and employee relations should give written summaries of both sides of the issue to the appropriate administrative vice-president of the department(s) involved for review and resolution. The administrative vice-president should render a verbal and written decision to the employee within three (3) working days after having received all pertinent data on the case. If, at this level, the employee is still unhappy with the decision rendered, he or she may appeal the decision to the president of the facility. The president should review the grievance and render a FINAL verbal and written decision to the employee within three (3) working days of receipt of the case.

7. *Employee service program (E.S.P.)* This is a counseling service for employees designed to resolve personal difficulties such as marital conflicts, unhealthy family relationships, substance abuse, depression, problems on the job, stress, emotional crisis, legal concerns, and financial worries. E.S.P. first helps the troubled person define the problem and then assists in deciding how best to resolve it. This may involve a few discussions. In some complex situations a referral to some other source of help may be necessary. E.S.P. can also aid the employee whose job performance is suffering; when the employee's performance and effectiveness are seriously deteriorating, the supervisor may recommend E.S.P. as a way of resolving the cause of the problem. E.S.P. should be strictly confidential and easy to use.

8. *Idea box.* Boxes for ideas, comments and suggestions (not needing immediate review and attention) should be located in conspicuous places. Ideas should be collected twice each month and then forwarded to the appropriate department heads or managers for review and response. The bulletin boards should be used to post responses. Complex or policy-related ideas or questions may take an extended time for a reply. If a more rapid response is necessary, the Action Needed Now process should be used.

9. *Meeting with management.* Weekly informal breakfasts or dinners should be held by a member of the management team for eight or ten

employees selected on a rotating basis from various departments. Invitations for attendance should be provided at least one week in advance. Issues, problems, and suggestions discussed at the sessions should be recorded by the attending administrator, protecting whenever possible the anonymity of employees. Follow-up action should be taken and communicated to each employee attending, and copies of the minutes with replies should be posted on the bulletin boards.

10. *Personnel department answering service.* Normal hours of personnel department offices are usually Monday-Friday, 8:00 a.m.-5:00 p.m. Employees on all shifts, though, sometimes need to ask questions about wages, benefits, or other matters managed by the personnel department. A 24-hour answering service phone extension should be made available to all employees to make it convenient to ask questions and receive a prompt reply. The tape should be checked at the start of each working day and an initial response given to the employee either in writing or by phone.

The importance of participative management is paramount. Fiscal constraints and tougher competition brought about by the changes in Medicare reimbursement and other mandated health care finance legislation will force some facilities to close, merge with other institutions, or join multi-institutional systems. The successful health care facility of the coming decade must address such problems as staffing, productivity, job security, and economics openly and honestly, which means that human resource managers will need to spend a lot of time developing and monitoring participative management programs for the institution. Participative management, in order to work well, must be backed by formal as well as informal policies attesting to management's belief in the process.

Participative management should be a major part of all personnel programs. The best way of finding out how and where employees want to participate is through a morale survey. Morale surveys can give management valuable information on how employees feel about participative management.

CHAPTER 17

Understanding Morale Survey Data

WHAT IS A MORALE SURVEY?

Morale! The French would call it "esprit de corps" or the spirit of the group--a force so powerful that it can motivate unexpected human endeavor and create a sense of genuine satisfaction. Sociologists might refer to it as a collective opinion; psychologists might view it as group attitude. The athlete, dramatic artist, or business person might simply reduce the concept to "team spirit." There is agreement, however, that whatever it is called it is not merely important --it is essential. It is that subtle factor that, when missing or in short supply, leads to dissatisfaction, disagreement, criticism and complaint, human friction and conflict that results in opposition and formal confrontation. When morale is found in abundance, there is cooperative endeavor reflecting harmony, mutual support, encouragement, and inspiration.

Morale itself is not action but readiness of a group to act. Knowing the morale of that group, one can predict expected behavior of that group. Morale is reflected in the opinions, whether expressed or held back by the group--opinions that result from a combination of thought plus feeling to reflect each person's viewpoint. Emotionalized rationalizations can also be called attitudes--based not necessarily on fact but on a point of view that may reflect either reality or bias.

This suggests that morale, once measured, must be carefully interpreted to separate the thought from the emotion and to identify the facts. If morale is consistent with fact and is positive, there is no problem. If morale is consistent with fact that is negative, there is a problem that must be identified and resolved, ideally through common understanding and effort aimed at corrective action. When morale is inconsistent with fact and is in error, there is the need for information or exposure to new insights to modify the feelings, along with a reconstruction of thoughts to create positive morale, which would be made evident by common understanding coupled with common acceptance of the facts as they are.

What someone thinks and feels will determine how he or she will act or respond. Negative morale may equal negative actions and responses disruptive or destructive to the objectives of the endeavor. Positive morale restores positive opinions, reflecting one's own thoughts and feelings, which often spill over to shade or color other situations in more positive terms. People who feel good about their working situations tend to overlook or minimize the tensions and frustrations that may creep into the conditions or relationships at work.

Morale assessment is, therefore, a tool to be used by management much as it uses other auditing tools. Management audits financial records, takes inventory of stock, evaluates employee performance, or seeks reappraisal of facilities--suggesting awareness of the need to have its resources in good form. Yet, one of the often overlooked resources is morale or attitude. A morale study, then, is a technique by which management can view its operations through the employees' eyes, with the employees' thoughts and feelings. Employees' evaluations of management and management practices and relationships can help determine the strengths and the weaknesses of the operation and, when properly interpreted, can define both group and individual problems. They provide information by which to pursue knowledgeable decisions and actions. They establish the data from which realistic priorities can be determined.

Employees react to what they think and not necessarily to a factual situation. In addition, a person's point of view often determines the impact of any attempted communication. Two different people can view the same situation from different points of view and logically determine different messages or conclusions. Such differences may disrupt the normal employee-employee relationships and, even more, the desired employee-employer relationships.

There is today a greater awareness that employees differ in their needs, value systems, beliefs or philosophies, expectations, and degrees of commitment. In a sense, these reflect various dimensions of different points of view that may lead to differences of opinion and eventually a disturbance to or disruption of desired employee-employer relations. Management and the corporate organization may also have different needs, value systems, philosophies, expectations, and commitments; and such differences may actually provoke conflict rather than harmony.

The basic responsibility for the employee-employer relationship lies with management rather than the worker. From the first step of the person applying for employment, through the process of delegating specific authority to the worker to perform and pursue specific activities, and ending with the necessity for performance corrective discipline, corrective action or corrective communication, there tends to develop in the employee's mind a sense of dependency and of needing to protect his status with management. Therefore, in day-to-day relationships the employee tends to reflect to management, through his supervisor, what he believes management wants to hear. The good news is reported to the supervisor--not the bad news. This emphasis on the positive often deludes management into a false or unrealistic optimism.

A professionally conducted, formalized, and systematized employee attitude and morale survey is one means available to management to effectively ascertain the extent to which there is a commonality of understanding among the workers and between the workforce and management with regard to the essential elements in the employment relationship (see Exhibit 17-1). To what extent is there mutual understanding and acceptance of the wage and benefit program, the systems that provide job security, the effectiveness of the available procedures for settling grievances, the effectiveness of both the upward and downward flow of communications, the degree to which employees feel recognized and respected as individuals without discrimination or favoritism, the extent to which the em-

HUMAN RESOURCES SERVICES, INC.

VIEWPOINT©

EMPLOYEE ATTITUDE SURVEY

Exhibit 17-1.

How to Complete the Survey

1. All questions are completed by filling in ONE of the answer spaces (circles) to the right of the statement.

   EXAMPLE: I like the kind of work I do.

   If you are satisfied with your job, you would
   fill the answer space under Satisfied like this:

	5. Completely satisfied
	4. Satisfied
3. Neither satisfied nor dissatisfied	
	2. Dissatisfied
1. Completely dissatisfied	

   I like the kind of work I do.. ① ② ③ ● ⑤

2. This survey is designed for machine scoring. Your careful observance of these few simple rules would be appreciated.
   - Use only a No. 2 pencil.
   - Make heavy black marks that fill the circle.
   - Erase cleanly any answer you wish to change.
   - Make no stray marks of any kind.

   EXAMPLES

Improper Marks	Proper Mark
✓ ✗ ◐ ⊙	○ ○ ● ○

3. Note that different answer formats are used throughout the survey. For example you may be asked whether something occurs Quite a bit or Very little, whether something is Very important or Unimportant, or whether you are Satisfied or Dissatisfied, etc. Please be alert to these changes in answer formats.

4. Try to answer EVERY question frankly and thoughtfully. If a question DOES NOT APPLY TO YOU, leave it blank and go on to the next question.

5. Several of the questions in this survey ask about something in your "organization." This means the entire company, firm, or non-profit organization you work for.

Organization Code: ⟶

⓪ ⓪ ⓪ ⓪ ⓪ ⓪ ⓪ ⓪ ⓪	
① ① ① ① ① ① ① ① ①	
② ② ② ② ② ② ② ② ②	○ Full Time
③ ③ ③ ③ ③ ③ ③ ③ ③	
④ ④ ④ ④ ④ ④ ④ ④ ④	
⑤ ⑤ ⑤ ⑤ ⑤ ⑤ ⑤ ⑤ ⑤	○ Part Time
⑥ ⑥ ⑥ ⑥ ⑥ ⑥ ⑥ ⑥ ⑥	
⑦ ⑦ ⑦ ⑦ ⑦ ⑦ ⑦ ⑦ ⑦	
⑧ ⑧ ⑧ ⑧ ⑧ ⑧ ⑧ ⑧ ⑧	
⑨ ⑨ ⑨ ⑨ ⑨ ⑨ ⑨ ⑨ ⑨	

Exhibit 17-1, cont.

In this section, mark the answer for each question that corresponds to your situation. For example, if you are 30 years old, mark answer #2 for Question #1.

1. Age:
   Under 25 .... ○
   25-34 .... ○
   35-44 .... ○
   45-54 .... ○
   55 and over .... ○

2. Sex:
   Female .... ○
   Male .... ○

3. Number of years with the organization:
   Less than 1 year .... ○
   1 to 5 years .... ○
   6 to 10 years .... ○
   11 to 20 years .... ○
   21 years and over .... ○

4. Number of years in your present position:
   Less than 1 year .... ○
   1 to 5 years .... ○
   6 to 10 years .... ○
   11 to 20 years .... ○
   21 years and over .... ○

5. Amount of formal education:
   1-12 years .... ○
   High school graduate .... ○
   Some college .... ○
   College graduate .... ○
   Post Baccalaureate Degree education .... ○

6. What is your current pay schedule:
   Hourly .... ○
   Salaried, non-exempt .... ○
   Salaried, exempt .... ○

7. Number of people you directly supervise:
   None .... ○
   1 to 3 .... ○
   4 to 7 .... ○
   8 to 15 .... ○
   16 and over .... ○

The following questions are to be answered using the number associated with the choice that comes closest to your own feelings.

> **5. A great deal, or to a great extent**
> 4. Quite a bit
> **3. Somewhat**
> 2. Very little
> **1. Not at all, or none**

8. Are the people you work with
   friendly and helpful? .... ① ② ③ ④ ⑤

9. Does your job require you to
   perform a number of very
   different activities? .... ① ② ③ ④ ⑤

10. Does this organization encourage
    you, or provide you the
    opportunity to improve your
    professional knowledge or job skills?..... ① ② ③ ④ ⑤

11. Do you feel personally responsible
    for the results of your own work?........ ① ② ③ ④ ⑤

12. How much information do you
    get from other people about
    whether you are doing a good or
    bad job? .... ① ② ③ ④ ⑤

13. Does your job make the best use
    of your own particular skills
    and abilities?........................... ① ② ③ ④ ⑤

14. Considering the type of work you
    do, are your physical working
    conditions comfortable? .... ① ② ③ ④ ⑤

15. Do you feel that this organization
    is a good place to work? .... ① ② ③ ④ ⑤

16. How adequate is the orientation
    and on-the-job training of
    new employees? .... ① ② ③ ④ ⑤

17. Are the people in your work
    group encouraged to work
    together as a team? .... ① ② ③ ④ ⑤

18. Does your organization make the
    best use of new or improved work
    methods or other technical
    advances? .... ① ② ③ ④ ⑤

19. Is the information you receive
    from other people, work groups,
    and/or shifts adequate? .... ① ② ③ ④ ⑤

PLEASE TURN THE PAGE

Exhibit 17-1, cont.

The following questions are to be answered using the number associated with the choice that comes closest to your own feelings.

5. A great deal, or to a great extent
    4. Quite a bit
      3. Somewhat
        2. Very little
          1. Not at all, or none

20. Are personnel policies (e.g., discipline, terminations, time off for personal emergencies, etc.) in this organization clearly defined? .... ① ② ③ ④ ⑤

21. Do you feel that assignments of shifts or working hours are fair? .... ① ② ③ ④ ⑤

22. Is your supervisor friendly and helpful? .... ① ② ③ ④ ⑤

23. How much of your job effort is lost or is not productive because of things in the organization over which you have no control? .... ① ② ③ ④ ⑤

24. Do you feel that this organization has reasonable goals and objectives? .... ① ② ③ ④ ⑤

25. Do you feel that the managers of your organization are concerned about accomplishing the organization's goals? .... ① ② ③ ④ ⑤

26. Are you fairly paid for the work you do? .... ① ② ③ ④ ⑤

27. Compared to other similar organizations in the community, is this organization considered to be a desirable place to work? .... ① ② ③ ④ ⑤

28. Do you always know exactly what to do in order to do your job properly? .... ① ② ③ ④ ⑤

29. How much cooperation is there among the members of your work group? .... ① ② ③ ④ ⑤

30. How much does **your job** require or permit you the opportunity to learn new skills? .... ① ② ③ ④ ⑤

31. Is the supervision you receive on the job helpful to you in performing your work? .... ① ② ③ ④ ⑤

5. A great deal, or to a great extent
    4. Quite a bit
      3. Somewhat
        2. Very little
          1. Not at all, or none

32. Do you feel that there is good cooperation between your department and other departments? ..... ① ② ③ ④ ⑤

33. Does your supervisor have sufficient job knowledge to make decisions about your work? .... ① ② ③ ④ ⑤

34. Do you feel that your work is personally rewarding in and of itself? .... ① ② ③ ④ ⑤

35. How often do the higher level managers of your organization come through your work area? .... ① ② ③ ④ ⑤

36. Do you feel that job promotions in this organization are fair, objective, and impartial? .... ① ② ③ ④ ⑤

37. Is the management of this organization genuinely concerned about the employees? .... ① ② ③ ④ ⑤

38. Does too much information come to you through the "grapevine" rather than through proper channels? .... ① ② ③ ④ ⑤

39. Does this organization make a real effort to help employees improve themselves? .... ① ② ③ ④ ⑤

40. Do you have to spend too much time, effort, or money getting to and from work? .... ① ② ③ ④ ⑤

41. Do you have enough authority to accomplish the work that is expected of you? .... ① ② ③ ④ ⑤

42. All in all, how well does your job measure up to what you thought it would be when you took it? .... ① ② ③ ④ ⑤

43. Does your job give you an opportunity to do the things you do best? .... ① ② ③ ④ ⑤

44. Do you think that the people in other departments who you have to depend on are doing a good job? ...... ① ② ③ ④ ⑤

45. Does this organization encourage the employees to suggest ways of improving work methods? .... ① ② ③ ④ ⑤

Exhibit 17-1, cont.

5. **A great deal, or to a great extent**
    4. Quite a bit
    3. Somewhat
    2. Very little
    1. Not at all, or none

46. Does your job make a positive contribution to your overall happiness? .... ① ② ③ ④ ⑤

47. Do you feel that hard work is worthwhile considering the way your future with the organization looks now? .... ① ② ③ ④ ⑤

48. Are the things that happen in the organization important to you? .... ① ② ③ ④ ⑤

49. To what extent do you **prefer** a job that requires you to perform a number of very different activities? ...... ① ② ③ ④ ⑤

50. To what extent do you **prefer** a job where you always know exactly what to do in order to do your job properly? .... ① ② ③ ④ ⑤

51. To what extent do you **prefer** a job that requires you to work at a constant fast pace? .... ① ② ③ ④ ⑤

52. To what extent do you **prefer** a job that requires your complete attention or concentration? .... ① ② ③ ④ ⑤

53. To what extent do you **prefer** a job that requires or provides you with the opportunity to learn new skills? ...... ① ② ③ ④ ⑤

54. To what extent do you **prefer** a job in which you receive a great deal of information from other people about whether you are doing a good or bad job? .... ① ② ③ ④ ⑤

55. To what extent do you **prefer** a job where you feel personally responsible for the results of your work? .... ① ② ③ ④ ⑤

In the section below are listed several aspects of your job. Please indicate the importance of each of these for your overall job satisfaction. This can be done by selecting one of the five choices below:

    5. **Very important**
    4. Important
    3. Neither important nor unimportant
    2. Unimportant
    1. Very unimportant

56. Promotions .... ① ② ③ ④ ⑤

57. Co-workers .... ① ② ③ ④ ⑤

58. Supervision .... ① ② ③ ④ ⑤

59. Pay .... ① ② ③ ④ ⑤

60. Opportunity for additional training .... ① ② ③ ④ ⑤

61. Employee Benefits...................... ① ② ③ ④ ⑤

62. Organization's policies and goals .... ① ② ③ ④ ⑤

63. Supervisor's evaluations of your performance .... ① ② ③ ④ ⑤

64. Opportunity for transfer to another job or another department .... ① ② ③ ④ ⑤

The following questions are to be answered using the number associated with the choice that comes closest to your own feelings.

    5. **Almost always**
    4. Often
    3. Sometimes
    2. Seldom
    1. Almost never

65. How often do you leave work with a good feeling of accomplishment about the work you did that day? .... ① ② ③ ④ ⑤

66. Does your job require you to work at a constant, fast pace? .... ① ② ③ ④ ⑤

67. Does your job require your complete attention or concentration?.............. ① ② ③ ④ ⑤

68. Are enough people available in your work group to accomplish the necessary work load? .... ① ② ③ ④ ⑤

69. Do you often get conflicting orders or instructions and, as a result, often don't know what you are supposed to do? .... ① ② ③ ④ ⑤

70. Is the communication between the members of your work group good? ...... ① ② ③ ④ ⑤

Exhibit 17-1, cont.

The following questions are to be answered using the number associated with the choice that comes closest to your own feelings.

5. Completely satisfied
4. Satisfied
3. Neither satisfied nor dissatisfied
2. Dissatisfied
1. Completely dissatisfied

71. All in all, how satisfied are you with your job?.............................① ② ③ ④ ⑤

72. How satisfied are you that your pay reflects the effort you put into doing your work? ....① ② ③ ④ ⑤

73. How satisfied are you with the work performance of the people you work with (or those you supervise if you are a supervisor)? ....① ② ③ ④ ⑤

74. If you learn the skills needed for some other job in the organization, how satisfied are you that you would be able to transfer to that new job? ....① ② ③ ④ ⑤

75. How satisfied are you with the difference in pay between new employees and experienced employees doing the same job?...............① ② ③ ④ ⑤

76. Compared to other similar organizations in the community, how satisfied are you with the benefit package? ....① ② ③ ④ ⑤

77. How satisfied are you with this organization's personnel policies (e.g., discipline, terminations, time off for personal emergencies, etc.)? ....① ② ③ ④ ⑤

78. How satisfied are you that the work load in your work group is evenly and fairly distributed?........................① ② ③ ④ ⑤

79. How satisfied are you that the benefits you receive (e.g., hospitalization insurance, vacation, etc.) are adequate? ....① ② ③ ④ ⑤

80. How satisfied are you with your future prospects for promotion? ....① ② ③ ④ ⑤

81. Are you satisfied that the evaluation of your job performance by your supervisors is objective, fair, and impartial? ....① ② ③ ④ ⑤

82. How satisfied are you with the job promotions you have received to date? ....① ② ③ ④ ⑤

SUPPLEMENT A

83 ① ② ③ ④ ⑤   92 ① ② ③ ④ ⑤
84 ① ② ③ ④ ⑤   93 ① ② ③ ④ ⑤
85 ① ② ③ ④ ⑤   94 ① ② ③ ④ ⑤
86 ① ② ③ ④ ⑤   95 ① ② ③ ④ ⑤
87 ① ② ③ ④ ⑤   96 ① ② ③ ④ ⑤
88 ① ② ③ ④ ⑤   97 ① ② ③ ④ ⑤
89 ① ② ③ ④ ⑤   98 ① ② ③ ④ ⑤
90 ① ② ③ ④ ⑤   99 ① ② ③ ④ ⑤
91 ① ② ③ ④ ⑤   100 ① ② ③ ④ ⑤

SUPPLEMENT B

1 ① ② ③ ④ ⑤   11 ① ② ③ ④ ⑤
2 ① ② ③ ④ ⑤   12 ① ② ③ ④ ⑤
3 ① ② ③ ④ ⑤   13 ① ② ③ ④ ⑤
4 ① ② ③ ④ ⑤   14 ① ② ③ ④ ⑤
5 ① ② ③ ④ ⑤   15 ① ② ③ ④ ⑤
6 ① ② ③ ④ ⑤   16 ① ② ③ ④ ⑤
7 ① ② ③ ④ ⑤   17 ① ② ③ ④ ⑤
8 ① ② ③ ④ ⑤   18 ① ② ③ ④ ⑤
9 ① ② ③ ④ ⑤   19 ① ② ③ ④ ⑤
10 ① ② ③ ④ ⑤   20 ① ② ③ ④ ⑤

Exhibit 17-1, cont.

Human Resources Services, Inc.

Viewpoint©

Hospital Attitude Survey

The following questions are to be answered using the number associated with the choice that comes closest to your own feelings.

> 1 = not at all, or none
> 2 = very little
> 3 = somewhat
> 4 = quite a bit
> 5 = a great deal, or to a great extent

83. Do you feel that administrative policies and practices promote the most effective patient care?

84. Are you supported by your superiors when you have a problem with a patient or a member of a patient's family?

85. Do you feel that the hospital administrators will respond to your problems in a fair and understanding manner?

86. Are hospital policies clearly and accurately communicated?

87. Do you feel that the members of your work group have the skills and/or sufficient training to provide the best patient care?

88. Do you feel the employees of the hospital show an attitude of genuinely caring about the patients?

89. Do you receive the proper respect from people outside your immediate work group?

In the section below are listed several aspects of your working conditions. Please indicate your opinion of each of these using one of the five choices below.

> 1 = poor
> 2 = below average
> 3 = average
> 4 = above average
> 5 = excellent

90. Work space

91. Parking

92. Employee lounges

93. Availability of equipment

94. Maintenance of equipment

95. Employee food service

96. Meeting and training space

97. Availability of supplies

Exhibit 17-1, cont.

ADDITIONAL VIEWPOINTS

Now that you have filled in your questionnaire and have thought about all the different aspects of your job and the organization in general, what would you like to say in addition about the various areas listed? Please do not write on the back of this sheet and limit your responses to the lines provided.

Remember: This sheet will not be seen by anyone at the organization.

Pay, Benefits and Other Personnel-Related Policies

_____

_____

_____

_____

_____

_____

Supervision or General Opinions About Organization

_____

_____

_____

_____

_____

_____

All Other Policies or Working Conditions

_____

_____

_____

_____

_____

_____

Exhibit 17-1, cont.

ployee feels he can participate, grow, advance, and achieve within the present systems of personnel policies and practices? These are but a few of many critical concerns that must be measured and evaluated by modern management to provide and maintain a positive and productive work environment. Since management has the ultimate responsibility for the end results of the operation, then the responsibility to know and react to employee attitudes and morale becomes the responsibility of management.

WHEN AND WHY SHOULD A MORALE SURVEY BE TAKEN?

When and where discernible differences are identified from the ways in which management and employee view a given situation, management should ascertain whether that difference is based on actual fact or on misconstrued communication. Where the employee attitude or opinion is correct, there is the implied necessity for management action to correct the situation. On the other hand, where the employee attitude or opinion is in error or deviates from fact, there is the implied necessity for management to act by corrective communication. The final objective is that management and the workforce view similar situations from a similar point of view in order to promote both harmony and a team spirit.

Management and its workforce are not opponents. Each must fulfill its own separate and distinct responsibilities cooperatively to achieve the common interests of both parties while achieving the objectives of the corporate enterprise. Although this last thought may be idealistic, it is nevertheless a worthy objective for managerial pursuit. The evaluation of employee attitudes and morale becomes the single most effective means toward this objective.

INDICATIONS OF POOR OR DETERIORATING MORALE

Careful and continuing observation of the following factors in human relations can often indicate poor or deteriorating morale and employee attitudes.

- High or increasing labor turnover, particularly voluntary job desertion and planned resignations

- High or increasing or unusual absenteeism and use of sick leave

- Handicapped or difficult recruitment efforts resulting in negative employer image or reputation

- A sudden marked increase in grievances processed, or a total absence of grievances

- Instances of insubordination and increasing supervisory relations problems

- Low performance levels. Inefficient and ineffective work performance

- Increased frequency and severity of errors and accidents

- Evidence of employee group or collective behavior

- Low or reduced motivation; lethargic, apathetic or passive attitude

- Increased referral of employee problems by way of physicians, patients, hospital visitors, or other third parties

- Increased numbers and types of complaints filed with government investigatory agencies

- Receptivity for third-party representation through employee groups or associations, professional associations or organized labor unions.

MEANS OF MEASURING MORALE

- Labor turnover analysis--to determine final cause, contributing factors, sources by occupation or department, and comparative labor turnover rates

- Absentee analysis--frequency, intensity, frequency times intensity for absentee rate, source (occupation or department), and major causes

- Public image analysis--both general and public as well as special interest group reactions to specific image of hospital on basic employee-employer relations factors

- Analysis of grievance patterns--frequency and intensity by employee group or department, basis of grievance, reason for appeals, reaction to settlements, etc.

- Response to discipline and responsible supervisory practices

- Objective performance appraisal relating actual work performance to performance standards

- Employee attitude or morale surveys

- Exit interviews conducted by an objective party capable of using an in-depth interview technique to identify basic causes behind stated problems regarding the job, wages and benefits, the work environment, and supervisory relations.

AN ATTITUDE ASSESSMENT SURVEY
AS A MANAGEMENT TOOL

Since an attitude can be defined as a way of thinking and feeling about a person, place, issue, or thing, an Attitude Assessment Study must take into account both the rational or thought process of the employee and the emotionalism with which that rationale or thought process is treated. An attitude becomes important since it creates a predisposition to action. This is often not conscious action and tends to be immediate.

The fact that the employee thinks and feels as he does, and that he shares the thoughts and feelings of his co-workers, creates the strength or weakness of the morale environment and suggests either support or rejection of management by the workforce. The assessment of the attitude pattern of employee groups becomes, therefore, a meaningful tool if used prudently and cautiously by management. (See Exhibits 17-2 and 17-3).

Management also reflects a unique workforce. The members of the management team have thoughts and feelings about the operation that may or may not be different from those held by the employees. A critical concern in an Attitude Assessment Survey is to discern management attitudes and how they compare with those of other groups of employees. When there is general acceptance, support, or agreement between management and the workforce, there is no problem. When there is common agreement that something is wrong, deficient, or without merit, then there is at least an opportunity for cooperative and collaborative behavior to seek a remedy for the problem. But when there are differences of opinion, there arises the opportunity for opposition and confrontation.

It is not always that the management personnel, either top level or middle first-line, take the most positive position. One or more groups of employees may well have an even more positive attitude than the management groups. Upper and lower levels of management may not have the same point of view. It is further possible or even probable that there may be wide range in morale, with some groups presenting a hostile or near-hostile position while others express a euphoric attitude.

There are several principles that need to be recognized in attempting to deal with the massive amount of data contained in morale survey data:

MORALE - SURVEY PROCESS

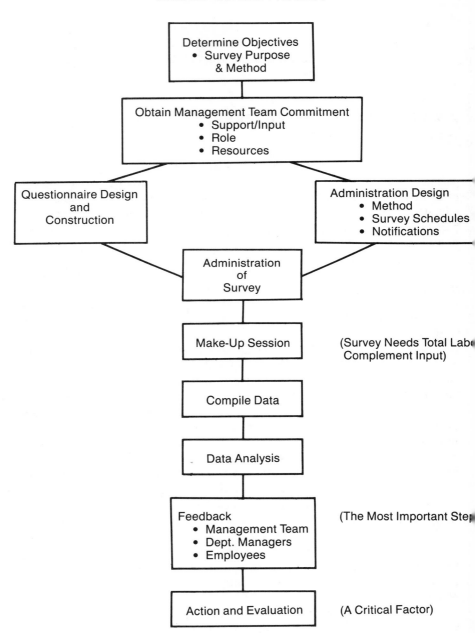

Exhibit 17-2.

... AND WHAT IS YOUR OPINION?

NOTE: What you think about your work, your work situation and your working relationships and conditions is important to us and important to you. A study of this type can help us to in turn help you by bringing forth improvements that are both possible and desirable. This study form has been designed to get as much information as easily as possible with little effort and time on your part. It is important, however, that you be frank and honest in your responses and be specific in your comments. This study form will not be reviewed by your employer, but will remain with the consulting staff and will result in a detailed report of findings and recommendations submitted to your employer. Your signature will not be required.

Exact Position Title: _____ Years of Service: _____

Department Title: _____ Cost Center: _____

Check One (1): I work day shift _____; evening shift _____; night shift _____; rotate _____

Check One (1): I work full time _____; part time_____; called as needed _____

I. Your Work Environment: - Circle the letter before each phrase to which you agree

A - A good place to work   B - Feel appreciated   C - Poorly organized
D - Often frustrated   E - Undersupervised   F - A friendly place

II. Your Work and Compensation: - Circle the letter before each phrase to which you agree

A - Could earn more elsewhere   B - Seniority counts   C - Often tiring
D - My work is rewarding   E - Overworked   F - Work is important
G - Paid equal to others   H - Lack fringe benefits   I - Just a job

III. Your Future: - Circle the letter before each phrase to which you agree

A - Opportunity to learn   B - Signs of progress   C - Plan to stay
D - Growth and advancement   E - Proud to work here.   F - Have a good future

SPECIFIC ISSUES

NOTE: For each of the issues listed circle the appropriate letter to indicate whether you strongly disagree (SD), disagree (D), are uncertain (?), agree (A), or strongly agree (SA). In the column marked "Description of Problem" indicate, if possible, why you are uncertain or do not agree.

STATEMENT OF ISSUE	RESPONSE	DESCRIPTION OF PROBLEM
1. My immediate supervisor generally tries to keep me well informed in advance.	SD D ? A SA	
2. Regular conferences held with my supervisor are generally helpful.	SD D ? A SA	
3. My present wages and fringe benefits are comparable to what I would expect to earn elsewhere.	SD D ? A SA	
4. I believe that I do properly understand the established procedure for handling complaints or grievances.	SD D ? A SA	
5. My work has been assigned within the scope of my present abilities.	SD D ? A SA	
6. I feel generally secure in that my present job will last.	SD D ? A SA	
7. I feel I can communicate upward to my supervisor, department head or even top administration.	SD D ? A SA	
8. Discipline is administered fairly when it is needed.	SD D ? A SA	

Exhibit 17-2, cont.

STATEMENT OF ISSUE	RESPONSE					DESCRIPTION OF PROBLEM
9. My wages have been adjusted satisfactorily in relation to the cost of living.	SD	D	?	A	SA	
10. I would have no hesitancy to voice my complaints directly with my supervisor.	SD	D	?	A	SA	
11. My co-workers and I have been assigned a balanced share of the total workload.	SD	D	?	A	SA	
12. Management systems such as the personnel policies, wage plan, my job description, my supervisor relationships all give me a real sense of security.	SD	D	?	A	SA	
13. I feel my voice is heard and respected in work area decisions.	SD	D	?	A	SA	
14. My supervisor and I have the same understanding of the work I am to do.	SD	D	?	A	SA	
15. My wages have kept pace with my increased productivity.	SD	D	?	A	SA	
16. I believe I could use the grievance procedure without any fear of resentment or reprisal.	SD	D	?	A	SA	
17. I received adequate orientation and job instruction training to undertake the tasks assigned me.	SD	D	?	A	SA	
18. I feel I would be promoted if my performance and qualifications were satisfactory.	SD	D	?	A	SA	
19. I feel the formal communications keeps me better informed than the grapevine.	SD	D	?	A	SA	
20. I feel my supervisor is adequately supported by higher management regarding decisions to solve our work problems.	SD	D	?	A	SA	
21. My fringe benefits have a value of an additional 20% to 25% over my basic wage.	SD	D	?	A	SA	
22. Grievances filed through the grievance system are fairly and objectively settled.	SD	D	?	A	SA	
23. I feel there are adequate continuing education and training programs to properly qualify me to fulfill my work requirements.	SD	D	?	A	SA	
24. My present work provides opportunity for both growth and advancement and promotion.	SD	D	?	A	SA	

Exhibit 17-2, cont.

STATEMENT OF ISSUE		RESPONSE				DESCRIPTION OF PROBLEM

25. My advice or recommendations are often sought.

SD   D   ?   A   SA

26. My immediate supervisor generally responds satisfactorily to my problems.

SD   D   ?   A   SA

27. As a general rule it would seem that there is equal pay for equal work.

SD   D   ?   A   SA

28. I feel top management wants to know my grievances so they can work to solve them.

SD   D   ?   A   SA

29. Work schedules seem to be determined fairly.

SD   D   ?   A   SA

30. When I have reached my maximum wage for my present work I can still expect economic advancement through promotion opportunities.

SD   D   ?   A   SA

31. Because sound decisions are made by top management there is little money wasted.

SD   D   ?   A   SA

32. My supervisor would encourage me to accept a transfer or promotion even at the risk of disturbing present work unit staffing.

SD   D   ?   A   SA

33. Personnel policies are satisfactorily revised and updated to meet current employee needs.

SD   D   ?   A   SA

34. The wage I earn is appropriate for the work I perform.

SD   D   ?   A   SA

35. There is no conflict between my goals and the present objectives of the hospital.

SD   D   ?   A   SA

36. I find the evaluation of my performance to be helpful.

SD   D   ?   A   SA

37. I have not felt insecure because of continuing improvements in the efficiency and cost reductions.

SD   D   ?   A   SA

38. I find that I am in general agreement with the philosophy that guides the decisions and actions of top management.

SD   D   ?   A   SA

39. My supervisor is able to respond appropriately to human relations problems.

SD   D   ?   A   SA

40. Based on my understanding of the system by which wages are determined I believe it to be fair and adequate.

SD   D   ?   A   SA

41. If I had a serious unresolved complaint I feel it would be to my best interest to have a face-to-face meeting with my department director or a member of the administrative staff.

SD   D   ?   A   SA

Exhibit 17-2, cont.

STATEMENT OF ISSUE	RESPONSE	DESCRIPTION OF PROBLEM
42. The performance evaluation system is properly used.	SD D ? A SA	
43. I can count on top management giving my immediate supervisor the support that is needed so that we can make necessary improvements in our work situation.	SD D ? A SA	
44. My supervisor often follows my recommendations.	SD D ? A SA	
45. Changes made this past year in the personnel program show continuing improvement and progress.	SD D ? A SA	
46. Most of the time the employee and the immediate supervisor work well together as a team.	SD D ? A SA	
47. I have a good sense of security based on my understanding of the present retirement program.	SD D ? A SA	
48. The present sick leave policy is adequate to give me a sense of economic security.	SD D ? A SA	
49. I have been made fully aware of the present personnel policies and practices.	SD D ? A SA	
50. This hospital at present enjoys a good reputation in the community which contributes to my pride and satisfaction.	SD D ? A SA	

A. List the six conditions or situations that you like least in your present work situation:

1. _____ 2. _____ 3. _____

4. _____ 5. _____ 6. _____

B. List the six conditions or situations that you like best in your present work situation:

1. _____ 2. _____ 3. _____

4. _____ 5. _____ 6. _____

C. What value do you think will come from this study?

_____

_____

GENERAL COMMENTS:

Date _____   No Signature Necessary

Exhibit 17-2, cont.

DIMENSIONS USUALLY MEASURED	QUESTIONS ARE DESIGNED TO INCLUDE EACH OF THE FOLLOWING
1. Job satisfaction	Challenge Motivation Participative aspects
2. Job mobility/advancement	Opportunity to transfer Opportunity to advance
3. Administration	Effectiveness Interest in employees Responsiveness Accessibility Visibility
4. Supervision	Effectiveness/quality Leadership Management skills Visibility Accessibility Responsiveness
5. Communications	Among departments From administration Effectiveness
6. Personnel policies	Understanding Fairness and consistency
7. Job security	Perceived job security
8. Salary/wages	External competitiveness Internal equity Perceptions
9. Benefits	Overall program
10. Working conditions	Equipment Appearance/cleanliness of work area Safety
11. Work relationships	Working together Cooperativeness Friendliness Morale
12. Job demands	Workloads/assignments Work pace Hours of work Job pressure

Exhibit 17-3.

13. Productivity	Utilization Efficiency/effectiveness Time wasted Absenteeism Cost containment
14. Participation	Organization decisions Department decisions Identity with facility
15. Performance evaluation	Helpful to development Measures of job performance Objective/subjective Fairness and consistency
16. Patient Care	Quality Confidence Community perception
17. Training/orientation	Adequacy Instructions Supportiveness

18. Caring environment	Rights, privacy and dignity of
	  patients
	Attitude towards public,
	  fellow employees
	Courteousness
	Responsiveness

19. Quality assurance	Problem identification Problem solving
20. Etc. (open dimension)	Open area for general comments

Exhibit 17-3, cont.

- Workers tend to resist and resent that which is imposed upon them, whereas they tend to commit themselves to and be motivated by that which they propose. This suggests the need for some means of participation of the employee group with management in a common effort to resolve issues.

- Management is not the master and the workforce the servant; in reality, they must serve each other's needs. The needfulness or relevancy of management is immediately apparent in a survey. The real sense of serving is in the essence of development. Management does not tend to the workforce--management develops the workforce.

- Imperfections observed become insecurities that are covered up--and insecurities harbored often become insults or criticisms that are hurled. In a sense, management provides through a morale study a special opportunity for the employee to ''attack.'' It is absolutely crucial that management forego the opportunity to ''attack back.'' The normal temptation is to become defensive by directing criticism to the employee. Management must be mature enough to recognize that a morale study often is limited to an expression of how the employee feels and thinks, but not necessarily why. The follow-through from such a study is aimed at discovery of the why and agreement as to what to do about it.

An Attitude Assessment or Morale Study, therefore, is a tool. It focuses attention on the areas of strength or weakness, but it requires action if it is to be a meaningful tool and one which can be used again and again in the future. Management should want to be the first informed when employees have problems. Successful use of a morale survey will often establish that degree of confidence in the minds of employees that management is a friend and is responsive to the real needs of the institution and its workforce.

CONFRONTATION WIDENS DIFFERENCES

Confrontation widens differences. A union organizing effort is a confrontation between employees, through a representative and management. Just as members of opposing political parties must emphasize their differences on basic issues, so too in a labor organizing effort--which is intended to climax in an election with management and the union vying for the employee's vote--differences rather than similarities are emphasized. Every management mistake during the campaign or in the recent past is vividly portrayed to the employee.

It is important to separate practice from expectation and to widen this difference until the employee can vote his informed conscience. The vote itself separates winners from losers and climaxes an understanding of differences in the parties.

When the union wins, these differences are important to prepare the negotiating team for open confrontation through the collective bargaining negotiations as well as to educate employees about the process and their need to ratify the final agreement. When management wins, employees frequently begin fearing revenge or retaliation from their supervisors for their union activities and sympathies. Fear and insecurity also frequently replace an appreciated relationship and confidence in management.

A morale survey offers management a unique opportunity to both qualitatively and quantitatively measure the real, not the alleged, differences in attitudes, points of view, or opinions on basic factors in the management-employee relationships.

The data revealed by a morale survey enable management to reestablish and maintain credibility where it has been damaged by the union campaign. Such a study can assure employees that management now knows, understands, and can accept the employee's point of view on important relationship issues. By stated and dated action plans effectively executed on a timely basis, management can move either with corrective action where the problem is real or with corrective communication where the employee's opinion is not well-founded, and then through appropriate communication can gain recognition by the employee that management has responded. To know it, to say it, to do it, and to get credit for it are essential aspects of the process of gaining and keeping credibility.

A morale survey provides information by which management can determine what should be done (the action); who should do it (the employee, the supervisor, administration, or a combination); when it should be done (the clock time or calendar) date (when results can be expected); how it should be done (procedures and methods and adherence to established practices, philosophies and standards); and where it should be done (the whole institution, a department, a unit, a shift, or perhaps just a single job). Why it should be done is often self-evident when the contrast between management's point of view and the employee's point of view is understood.

Commonality of interest, objective, and attitude is often essential to build harmony and a sense of teamwork. Morale data provide a basis for the employee to join with management in a common undertaking to resolve differences that may exist in fact or fancy between management and the employee.

Each survey is unique. Perhaps the greatest consistency is the inconsistency in replies by groups to certain questions. In dealing with a series of Attitude Assessment Surveys, one quickly recognizes that the old stereotyped beliefs are quickly set aside. It is not true that all dietary workers believe they are underpaid. It is not true that all nurses are happy and derive a great sense of satisfaction out of their state of dedication. It is not true that if employees earn a sufficient wage, their morale is good. It is not true that employees merely want to report to duty, do their work, and be left alone. It is also not true that management alone sets the tone of the operation that influences a general level of morale. Each study is unique as each worker is unique, and the differences are important in understanding morale.

In a careful review, by the authors of 61 separate Attitude Assessment Surveys conducted in health care facilities during 1978 and 1979 in 17 states representing all regions of the U.S.A. and reflecting the attitudes of 66,871 paid staff, a number of interesting worker moods and attitudes emerged. The following information is presented not as normative data but as the result of a careful assessment of possible patterns and trends in employee-management relations that can help to shed a sense of awareness of why some managers are successful and others are not.

PREDOMINANT THRUSTS OF MORALE CONCERNS

Several factors emerge as predominant employee morale concerns, but it is essential to recognize that predominance does not mean consistency. These few factors are not necessarily consistent from one study to the next, one employer to the next, or even one employee to the next within the same study in the same center of employment.

1. *Wages* are not always the primary area of concern, but employees do watch both their paychecks and management's actions regarding improvement of those paychecks. As a result, employees become highly sensitive to the management decisions that require expenditures of funds --funds that could have been redirected to the wage or benefit package, but because of management's decision have been spent on something else.

   Wages have emerged as important enough to draw the unsolicited reaction of 70 to 85 percent of the average workforce. Health care employees' concerns center around a general belief that their present rate of pay is inadequate for the level of responsibility that must be assumed when one works for a health care facility, the amount of preparation and experience required for performance, and the general level of expected productivity. The employees further believe that increased responsibility, extra workload, or growth and advancement within the job justifies a far greater recognition of merit or increased productivity than management has been willing to grant.

   There is a strong belief among health care workers that little external equity exists in health care wages. Further, there is little confidence in internal equity and, as a result, minimal confidence in the system by which wages are determined.

2. *Career mobility* runs a close second to wages as a morale factor to most groups of health care employees. Nearly 80 percent of health care workers want to have a more promising career future than they currently believe they have (in spite of the continuing education opportunities provided by health care facilities), not only to keep them abreast of developments in their current fields but also to expand their knowledge and skills as a necessary forerunner to promotion.

As important as these two issues are, when the conditions satisfy the economic and career needs of the employee, they become almost unidentifiable concerns. In other words, when wages and opportunities are satisfactory, they become unimportant. It is only their lack of satisfaction that causes them to emerge as important attitude problems.

UNEXPECTED ISSUES AND TRENDS

There are often elements of surprise in a morale study as management reads what employees want and how they feel about specific aspects of management's performance. Because they are unexpected, they often become particularly sensitive factors. What are these unexpected factors?

1. *Seniority* is a more important issue to the newer employee than it is to the long-term worker. If the newcomer believes that the employer treats with dignity and satisfaction the person and the loyalty of the long-term worker, there is an opportunity to gain a sense of confidence and commitment from that new worker.

2. There is a strong and openly expressed desire for more intensive and more consistent exercise of *discipline* by management over the workers who fail to abide by the work rules; who fail to complete assigned work; who fail to maintain schedules; who abuse sick leave; who do not foster harmony, cooperation, and mutual support. The good employee feels impinged upon by the lazy, incompetent, or indifferent employee. The worker merely present to pick up a paycheck does not have the respect of his co-workers. The co-workers then question why management does not exercise discipline so that such an individual does not interfere with the work, performance, schedules, or general environment of the cooperative and productive employees.

3. Most employees want to do a good job, believe they have done a good job, and therefore want their performance to be *evaluated* even more frequently. Employees want firsthand knowledge of their deficiencies so they can overcome them and regain the confidence of their supervisors and enjoy the benefits provided for the good performer. What employees do not want is destructive, personalized criticism. They do not want a performance evaluation that is viewed as a weapon in the hands of the supervisors. They want an instructive and constructive review of actual performance based on assignments of tasks, with identification of specific deficiencies and appropriate consultation to guide and assist the employee in growth, advancement, and improvement. Supervisors may view the performance evaluation as a burdensome chore. Employees often view that same performance evaluation as a benefit that management is obligated to provide. When provided with a sense of understanding, empathy, and compassion, the evaluation becomes a mutual benefit to the employee and the supervisor alike.

4. *Human dignity* is a vital factor to each person. Employees want to be identified, recognized, and appreciated. They want to know that someone cares--that management is concerned about employment conditions and is responsive to those that are deficient. Perhaps the most significant factor in an employee's total work environment is a caring and sensitive supervisor.

5. The *desire to be a partner,* to have a voice in advance of decision making, is a constantly increasing factor among employees. They think that if higher management respects the workers, it must give them opportunity to speak out on aspects of the work or the work environment on which they are the specialists. This issue becomes so acute in some instances that voice in the affairs of the work is viewed as a right, not a privilege or a new style of management.

6. The desire for a sense of *consistency,* singleness of purpose, togetherness, family community, or other such concepts, seems to express itself in the Attitude Assessment Surveys. Employees want to understand the philosophy and guiding principles that direct top management decisions and the consistency with which the philosophy and principles are observed. Similarly, they want to know the goals of the institution to determine the extent to which they are compatible with their own goals. As an example of this latter factor, most expansion programs, rather than creating a firm sense of security and protection, tend to be viewed as a major threat to the employees who feel overworked and short-staffed and who see the expansion program as meaning either increased workload and work responsibilities or a new center for work performance that will drain away some of the available productive hours of the present peer group.

7. *"Professionalism"* to some extent has replaced the term "dedication." There is a strong desire for professional attitudes, behavior, appearance, and language--and equal disdain for the employee who lacks the same. Professionalism stimulates interest in patient care, service to mankind, and mutual support; and it requires a sense of cooperative and collaborative behavior aimed at a commonality of purpose. It tends to substitute a collective interest for a private interest.

8. Perhaps one of the major surprises in a morale survey is the *ongoing frustration of employees who are in a collective bargaining unit* and under a collective bargaining agreement. The sense of unhappiness and dissatisfaction that stimulates interest in a collective approach to problem reduction apparently remains long after a contract is negotiated. Perhaps mutual respect, trust, confidence, harmonious relationships, effective

two-way communication, and realistic security are, in fact, nonnegotiable factors--in contrast to wages, benefits and rules, or regulations which are negotiable.

9. The worker wants the *supervisor* as a kind of friend. The supervisor is often viewed by higher levels of management as the first line of management but by the worker as the last rung of the workers' ladder. The employee wants competency, availability, a willing listener, an able communicator, a source for support, and a leader. The worker looks for expressed appreciation, a sense of caring and concern, and one able to respond effectively to recommendations, problems, and grievances. In those senses, the worker wants a friend.

These are some of the major desires that employees indicate that often seem to surprise management. Perhaps one more broad area that is surprising is the immediate impact of economic, social, and political issues on the workplace, causing reexamination of normal working factors and often resulting in a different sensitivity of morale.

MORALE ISSUES THAT REFLECT THE OUTSIDE ENVIRONMENT

Factors identified in Attitude Assessment Surveys that do not come from within the organization but reflect the outside influences of economics, politics, or society in general, frequently include the following:

1. Surprisingly, the insecurity presented by in-house *cost containment* programs is no major problem. The employee who must make continuous economic adjustments in his private life to keep abreast of the cost of living spiral seems appreciative of the need for the employer to do likewise. The employee views efficiency and cost containment efforts not as potential job threats, but as special sources of security that protect accrued benefits, ultimate retirement, and money available for future wage adjustments. It is not infrequent that the absence of such activities leads to insecurity.

2. For a decade, many sociologists and others have questioned whether *commitment* is still a possibility in society. The lack of commitment to tradition, values, authority, and social institutions has suggested that a sense of personal commitment is a sign of the past. Attitude Assessment Surveys belie this. Employees want to be assured not only that personal goals are consistent with those of the institution, but also that their personal philosophy is consistent with the philosophy that guides major in-

stitutional decisions. Many employees want to have a firm sense of pride in the employer. They want to believe their work is important. The reputation of the employer in the community is often a major factor contributing to a sense of job fulfillment. There is even resentment expressed by the majority for the minority who view their jobs as just jobs--a means to a paycheck and not an opportunity for service.

3. There is a high sensitivity among employees who feel left out and, as a result, are unaware of the real signs of progress in employee relations and patient care services. They want to be *informed* and to know the progress that is being made.

4. Responsiveness to new social issues can and does occur at any time. In these years of political debate over changes in health care finances and methods of health care delivery, health care employers can anticipate new and changing morale issues. Those new morale issues will reflect the pressures of the outside environment, and it will be important for management to identify those concerns and respond quickly.

THE HARD MORALE ISSUES

A wide range of special administrative problems is also revealed in Attitude Assessment Surveys. They are not problems that can be resolved in a wink or with a snap of the fingers. They require long planning and effort, and often involve collaborative effort between the employees and management if the problems are to be resolved at all. What are these hard issues?

1. The sense of being *overworked,* pressured, often tired, and generally short-staffed is a frequent employee concern. It directly challenges management's performance standards or productivity standards, and it requires an intense analysis and assessment of work activities including an understanding of procedures methodology and task purposes.

2. The question of *which co-workers become friends* is a somewhat new problem in morale. Once it was the peer group versus management, but today there appears not to be consistency of appreciation for all of one's peers. The problems of backstabbing, complaining, personal gossip, nonsupport, apathy, and other such factors tend to divide the employees as a group and further aggravate the problem of team building for management.

3. *New ideas of communication* have emerged at the very time that management is attempting to formulate new systems for information flow.

Employees no longer view in-house publications, administrative memos, letters, or bulletin board notices as communication. They say communication is an exchange of ideas and thus requires one-to-one contact or small group discussions. The employees have also added an important dimension that consequential communication is discussion based on topics of mutual interest and leads to a decision--and that that decision must lead to an action. This establishes the basis for the new push for participation.

4. The *commonality of purpose* or objective that leads to an interdependent relationship reflected by cooperative behavior becomes an important factor to employees. They question problems of interdepartmental conflict, intershift conflict, and interpersonal conflict.

5. The desire for a *visible and credible top leader* in administration has grown as a factor. People want to know and be known by that person. They want to know that this individual cares and is responsive to their needs. They believe that such a person must display respect for other people and as a result be easy to communicate with.

6. Somewhat crucial to the overall sense of confidence in a visible, credible leader is the need for a *system by which to reduce problems* and to resolve grievances. Most employees tend to believe that their leaders are already aware of the problem or the grievance and that continued existence is a sign that no one cares. There must, therefore, be effective communication throughout the procedure so that all understand the status of the issue and what must be resolved. The system must be built on confidence if it is to work at all. There is a strong desire today for self-representation even in a confrontation process.

7. A new sense of *positive human relations*--avoiding partiality, favoritism and discrimination and emphasizing recognition of human dignity through a personal identity that is appreciated--is a large and compact set of factors that boils down to the simple fact that people want to be treated as equals in an atmosphere of respect. The supervisor who needs to be "loved" rather than respected may appear to "play favorites." This victimizes both the supervisor and the "pet" and antagonizes all others outside the relationship. Obviously problems of sexism, racism, and nonequal treatment reflect a vintage of the past and should not be borne into the future.

8. *Employee benefits* have come to be viewed as a collateral wage and thus are to be as well-defined as the rate of pay. The part-time employee now not only wants but also feels entitled to a full proration of all fringe bene-

fits. Employees also seek equity with their neighbors and friends and thus they feel entitled to time-and-a-half pay for working holidays or weekends. The internal sense of equity suggests that the unused sick leave should be viewed as a benefit since the used day of sick leave was a benefit to someone. The personal day off becomes a more valuable holiday than many of the others that have been granted. The status of the longer vacation now suggests an earlier availability of the third and fourth week's vacation. There is, however, no point that establishes when enough is enough. There will always be new benefits to be sought and old benefits to be expanded.

9. Maintaining a sense of *job security* advocated and endorsed by management seems to be a major necessity. Employees tend not to get a lot of security from the wage system, their personnel policy handbook, or conferences with their supervisors. It is therefore vital to reexamine what management is doing to build the workers' sense of security and to establish a system that communicates job security.

10. The *need to overcome the "we"* and *"they"* within an organization is an absolute necessity. The need for absolute confidence in administration is as vital to the employee as the need for confidence in the supervisor is to the administrator. When an organization does not progress and win as a team, it tends to lose as individuals. In the long run this may in fact be the major purpose of an Attitude Assessment Study--to identify the difficulties that employees may find in establishing a true sense of team relationship with those who serve in the various levels of management.

"As the twig is bent so is the tree inclined." Similarly, as the attitudes of the employees are shaped, so is the behavior of the operation determined. A knowledge of negative attitudes as they exist affords management the opportunity to exercise corrective action where the attitudes have substance and corrective communication where they do not.

DEVELOPING AN ACTION PLAN

Survey results always make visible certain employee problems and concerns. It is a good idea to include in the action plan certain immediate, definite, concrete steps that management will take to make the employees' work more attractive and more important to the facility. The plan should be categorized into two sections--short-range goals/improvements and long-range goals on how the data obtained will be used to improve operations in the future. Employees really need to feel as though they've made a difference, that their participation in the survey was worthwhile, and that management listened and is doing something.

FEEDBACK PROCESS TO ALL EMPLOYEES

Providing feedback on results and sharing management action plans with employees is a crucial part of a morale survey. Employees look for action once the survey is completed. Having answered all the questions, they expect management to take an increased interest in their replies and do something about them. It is essential to report summarized survey results to employees. Summarized results can be communicated to employees in various ways--employee bulletin boards, publications, or various graphic or visual approaches, such as overhead transparencies and slide presentations. The most effective way, however, is through departmental meetings or roundtable discussions.

TIMING, CONTENT AND THE NLRB

Morale surveys are a standard diagnostic tool for management to detect basic dissatisfaction that could eventually lead to pro-union feelings, costly election campaigns, and possible unionization. In some circumstances, however, the legality of such surveys could be questioned, and their use could cause the results of an election in which the facility had been successful to be set aside. Most standard surveys contain questions that are rather unprejudicial and can easily pass a NLRB review. However, should the survey contain questions that pry into employees' feelings for or against unions, the NLRB could find it to be illegal.[1]

Management should not abandon the use of morale surveys simply because of possible pitfalls. It is advisable to clear surveys with legal counsel, especially when there is any indication of union activity or when the survey is to be given to employees who are already unionized.

FORMS AND METHODOLOGIES

There are many morale surveys on the market. Some are good and some are not. Using a poor survey can very well be worse than not using a survey at all. Exhibits 1, 2, and 3 outline a typical effective survey, the survey process to follow for a successful survey, and dimensions that a good survey should measure.

ENDNOTES

1. *Stanford University*, 240 NLRB No. 137 (1979).

CHAPTER 18

An Internal Professional Audit of the Personnel Function

Prudent administration would not question the necessity of an annual audit of its financial management records, insurances, and other fiscal matters. There should be equal participation for an audit of the personnel function within an institution. According to two experts in the field, "A personnel audit is much like a financial audit in purpose in that various personnel activities are examined using present and historical data."[1]

The purpose of the internal audit of the personnel department is to determine if the personnel function is being properly managed. The significance of some form of routine audit should be obvious. The major differences between one health care program and another tends to be a reflection of the competency and the attitudes of the workforce that prepares the products and provides the services that combine in the delivery of health care. What management does, therefore, to enhance various factors--selection, orientation, training, task development, communications, counseling, discipline and systems of reward, recognition and employee participation--becomes highly significant in the institution's ability to recruit and retain competent personnel and to enhance positive attitudes that reflect the concern and interest vital in adequacy of care of patients.

How can management therefore determine if personnel activities are being properly managed? It must first determine the objectives it desires to achieve in the personnel area and then design the audit process to determine the status of those objectives. The audit can include a number of areas but should include:

- Goals and objectives

- Caliber of personnel staff

- Personnel staffing data

- Human resource cost control

- Personnel policies

- Recruitment and selection

- Benefit administration

- Labor/employee relations

- Training and development

- Safety and employee health

- Wage and salary administration

- Records and controls

- Employee information and communication

There are several comprehensive self-administered personnel management audit systems now available in the market. A sample personnel audit checklist is presented in Exhibit 18-1. The most useful audit tool is one that "allows the institution to privately compare their responses to the current practice of other institutions of their size throughout the country."[2]

The auditor should be appointed by the chief executive officer. The person selected should be an experienced human resource specialist in the field of health care personnel administration.

The auditor has two sources for standards of measurement--the individual facility versus institutions its size throughout the country, and data accumulated within the personnel department.

The audit report should be given to the chief executive officer, who should use it in a positive way to identify areas that can be improved, establish specific new objectives, and increase the department's professional image and effectiveness. Most audits of this nature go a long way toward establishing the credibility of the human resource department with top management. The chief executive officer should use the report in the same manner as the fiscal auditor's report.

CALIBER OF PERSONNEL STAFF

The professionalism and competence of the personnel staff obviously have a direct impact on the output and effectiveness of the department. The absence of a reasonable proportion of high talent in personnel can be damaging to the institution. Incompetence in the department reduces the effectiveness of the personnel function in a score of subtle ways because personnel administration is a function where judgment, practical innovativeness, and "people sense" are key to success. Since personnel administration effectiveness depends to a large extent on line managers and other executives coming to the personnel office for assistance, it is imperative that they have confidence in the personnel staff. The audit process should include an assessment of the competency of the personnel staff.

There are a number of basic concepts and principles that affect employee wages and benefits, but that have generally been overlooked or ignored by health care managers in the struggle merely to keep pace with basic wages and the competition of the marketplace. A few of these fundamental principles are:

SAMPLE OF PERSONNEL AUDIT CHECKLIST

This audit is a basic inventory of the variables that influence
personnel administration operations. It is based on administrative
practices necessary for an effective and efficient human resource
management program. The questions are not comprehensive or all-
inclusive. The auditor should independently review, analyze, and
comment on each section.

Use of this audit will assist in identifying strengths and
weaknesses within the personnel administration area(s). A formal
written summary with specific recommendations should be prepared for the
chief executive officer (CEO).

The CEO should review the summary with the person responsible for
the personnel function, and outline a corrective course--set new goals
and/or modify existing goals.

	YES	NO	NA
A. GOALS AND OBJECTIVES			
The personnel program is based on goals and objectives established by the CEO	___	___	___
The goals are delineated in written form	___	___	___
The objectives have been reviewed by the CEO within the past year	___	___	___
The responsibilities and relationships of department heads for the personnel function are clearly defined	___	___	___
B. CALIBER OF PERSONNEL STAFF			
The person responsible for the personnel function has the necessary qualifications for the job	___	___	___
The department is adequately staffed	___	___	___
Members of the department are active in human resource professional associations	___	___	___
The department enjoys a good reputation within the institution	___	___	___
The staff members have all been properly trained for their jobs	___	___	___
There is a written plan of organization of the personnel function	___	___	___
C. PERSONNEL STAFFING DATA			
There is an authorized staffing plan for each department	___	___	___

Exhibit 18-1.

	YES	NO	NA
There is a position control plan	___	___	___
There is a system for Reduction in Force (RIF) and layoff	___	___	___
D. HUMAN RESOURCE COST CONTROL			
There is a system of personnel productivity based upon scientifically predetermined work measurement and standards	___	___	___
There is a policy requiring that the need for additional positions be justified by analysis	___	___	___
Job descriptions are used to assist in the assignment of functions to the appropriate employees	___	___	___
There is a system to provide a basis for evaluating individual employee performance	___	___	___
E. PERSONNEL POLICIES			
Personnel policies are comprehensive, well-written, and published in a manual	___	___	___
Employees are informed of changes in personnel policies at least 30 days in advance, and the changes are communicated to them in writing	___	___	___
Personnel policies are reviewed at least annually	___	___	___
The personnel policy manual provides the basis for administration of the facility's personnel program	___	___	___
Information in the employee handbook is abstracted from the personnel policy manual	___	___	___
F. RECRUITMENT AND SELECTION			
There is a centralized personnel function through which all applicants must pass	___	___	___
There is a specific person who is responsible for the overall employee recruitment function	___	___	___

Exhibit 18-1, cont.

	YES	NO	NA
The responsibility and authority pertaining to employee recruitment has been defined in writing	___	___	___
Department heads have been properly trained in interviewing techniques	___	___	___
The orientation program is reviewed to evaluate its effectiveness	___	___	___
The orientation program coordinates new employee indoctrination, job training, performance, and follow-up	___	___	___

G. BENEFIT ADMINISTRATION

There is an employee benefits program that is at least comparable to those offered by other area employers	___	___	___
The employee benefit program is reviewed at least annually	___	___	___
Employees are regularly informed of the various benefits provided and their annual dollar value	___	___	___

H. LABOR/EMPLOYEE RELATIONS

There is a committee of the governing board that concerns itself with labor relations	___	___	___
A formal employee grievance procedure is established and published in the employee handbook	___	___	___
The CEO keeps informed of the latest developments concerning labor and collective bargaining practices in the health field	___	___	___
The CEO is familiar with provisions of state and federal labor laws as they apply to health care institutions	___	___	___

I. TRAINING AND DEVELOPMENT

There is a planned program of employee training and development	___	___	___
Training objectives are related to departmental objectives	___	___	___

Exhibit 18-1, cont.

	YES	NO	NA
The annual budget includes allocation of specific funds to implement the training and development programs	___	___	___
There is a stated policy permitting selected personnel to attend workshops, institutes, and other educational programs at the expense of the facility	___	___	___
Employees who attend workshops and institutes are required to report on their experiences so others can benefit	___	___	___
Adequate facilities and equipment are provided for the conduct of training and educational programs	___	___	___

J. *SAFETY AND EMPLOYEE HEALTH*

There is an organized employee health service	___	___	___
There is a health record for each employee	___	___	___
The objectives of the employee health program are stated in writing	___	___	___
There is a designated physician in charge of the employee health service	___	___	___
Sufficient facilities are available for private interviews and examination of job applicants and employees	___	___	___
The employee health service includes an employee immunization program	___	___	___

K. *WAGE AND SALARY ADMINISTRATION*

There are written policies that guide the program of wage and salary administration	___	___	___
There is an established wage range showing minimum, maximum, and intermediate steps for each position	___	___	___
There is a formal procedure for periodic evaluation of employee performance	___	___	___

Exhibit 18-1, cont.

	YES	NO	NA
Department heads participate in a review of staffing plans for the forthcoming year	___	___	___
Department heads participate in the job evaluation program for their departments	___	___	___
Position evaluation includes the use of job specifications	___	___	___

L. *RECORDS AND CONTROLS*

	YES	NO	NA
There is a standard content for personnel records	___	___	___
There is a specific person in the facility who is responsible for maintaining the standard content of personnel records	___	___	___
There is an attendance record for each employee	___	___	___
There is a designated procedure for handling records of terminated employees	___	___	___
The department has a system for reporting data to the CEO	___	___	___

The facility uses the following Bureau of Labor Standard Formula for computing personnel turnover.

$$\frac{S \text{ (number of separations during the month)}}{M \text{ (Mid-month employment)}} \times 100 = T$$

(Mid-month employment is the number of employees on the payroll for the pay period ending on the day closest to the 12th of the month)

M. *EMPLOYEE INFORMATION AND COMMUNICATION*

The following methods of communication with employees are utilized.

	YES	NO	NA
House publication	___	___	___
Employee handbook	___	___	___
Payroll inserts	___	___	___
Bulletin boards	___	___	___
Suggestion award program	___	___	___
Grievance procedure	___	___	___

Exhibit 18-1, cont.

```
                                            YES      NO       NA

        Employee management meetings        ___      ___      ___

        Counseling services                 ___      ___      ___


MISCELLANEOUS AUDIT QUESTIONS

Date of last morale survey?        _____

Does the department conduct exit interviews?   _____

Does the department have access to labor counsel?   _____

Is there a system to monitor unemployment benefit claims?   _____

Is there a need for an automated personnel information
  system?   _____

Are EEO and Affirmative Action Plan documents current?   _____

Is there a system to monitor licensure/registrations?   _____

Is the concept of participative management visible within the
  department?   _____        The institution?   _____


NOTES AND COMMENTS
```

Exhibit 18-1, cont.

1. Wages tend to be viewed as a cost, not as an investment.

2. Wages tend to be used to purchase talent rather than to purchase performance. Even worse, and more frequent, they are used to purchase time.

3. Ultimately, wages must respond to the economic laws of supply and demand, so that inadequate wages tend to produce inadequate labor.

4. Health care facilities have failed to recognize that for cost control purposes, it is the work that must be controlled internally--not the price of labor, which is determined externally.

5. There is no one absolute and right system to determine wages.

6. Wages, when right, tend to be correct only in relationship so that there is both equity internally among the jobs within the health care facility and external equity between health care wages and those of competitive enterprises.

7. Benefits need to be viewed as collateral wages and must be as specifically defined as the rate of pay per hour or per unit of performance.

8. Recruitment tends to be based on the wage rates, whereas retention tends to be based on benefits.

9. Wages, if generally adequate, tend to fall to a secondary priority in the mind of the average health care worker.

10. Avoidance of internal distortions in normal economic relationships requires a formal, organized system of wage and benefit administration with pay grades, wage ranges, established wage policies, wage and benefit surveys, and performance appraisal.

BASIC ADMINISTRATIVE WAGE AND BENEFIT PROBLEMS FOR AUDIT CONSIDERATION

Although the statement "a worker is worthy of his hire" is apparently a simple one, it is difficult to determine today exactly what it means and how it can be applied. Administration now faces many problems that a few years ago did not exist.

1. More legal basis and precedents exist for setting or determining certain aspects of a wage program formerly left to the discretion of administration. Included are not only conditions under the equal pay provisions of the amendments to the Fair Labor Standards Act, but also the potential problems of comparable worth.[3]

2. New changing social attitudes place special pressures on administration to control health care costs either through cost containment or cost reduction efforts, while at the same time keeping employees out of poverty wage levels. This latter practice tends to be rejected when administratively pursued but accepted when negotiated through union collective bargaining.

3. Social justice applies pressure for increased rates of pay to the employees but lower health care costs for the patients.

4. Various views favor varied systems of wages, from the single rate system to multilevel wage plans.

5. Legal questions arise over cost-saving techniques such as compensatory time off in lieu of overtime payment, and volunteerism by employees.[4]

6. The question continues as to whether wages are intended to buy time, qualifications, performance, productivity, or status.

7. Cost-of-living adjustments have become a way of life, with lower scale employees stressing equal dollars and cents adjustments and higher employees demanding equal percentage adjustments. Tight money tends to create a diminishing return in cost-of-living adjustments for higher rated jobs.

8. Administration and governing boards want a voice in wage determinations while their role has been reduced to a responsive approval of outside pressures and influences.

9. Instead of budgets controlling wages or benefits, wages or benefits tend to control and drive budgets.

10. Time is needed to adapt to new economic conditions for health care facilities that have become relatively complex and inflexible.

11. Compaction in wages promotes new problems of incentive, recognition, and economic substitution.

12. Economics has become a vital part of the health care work environment.

13. Wages are no longer considered a flexible cost but a fixed rate of expense.

14. Economic laws now apply to the health care industry the same as to other business and industry, and include the law of supply and demand, the law of economic substitution, and the law of diminishing returns.

15. The struggle to survive under fiscal constraints and restrictive state controls has opened up a "bidding up" war by health care facilities in search of executives with positive performance track records. As health care institutions scramble for qualified executives, the remuneration process is becoming increasingly disorderly. There are few or no long-range compensation strategies in place. As the scramble increases, the disorderly situation will no doubt get worse before it gets better. How can health care facilities meet the marketplace realities yet properly control their spending for executive compensation?

HUMAN RESOURCE PHILOSOPHY

In a rapidly changing social-moral culture the human resource philosophy of a facility takes on a unique significance. Many of the new moralities have an impact within the institution. The belief by employees that they would support the philosophy of the operation if they fully understood it, suggests that there is an inadequate understanding of the organization's belief system. It is, therefore, recommended that the philosophy of the facility relative to human resource management matters be specifically defined and incorporated as part of the audit. Everyone should know the philosophy--not merely know where it is so he/she can look it up.

ENDNOTES

1. Robert L. Mathis and Gary Cameron, "Auditing Personnel Practices In Smaller-Sized Organizations," *Personnel Administration* (April 1981).

2. *Personnel/Human Resources Management Audit* (Wheeling, IL: Personnel and Professional Development, Inc., 1985).

3. 'Comparable worth' is a theory that whole classes of jobs are illegally undervalued because they are held by women. Proponents of comparable worth reason that job categories traditionally held by women have been undervalued simply because they are held by women, as compared to traditionally male jobs.

4. U.S. Department of Labor, Wage & Hour Division, ruling that an employment relation exists when a nonexempt employee volunteers his/her services at the hospital in which he/she is employed outside his/her regular working hours, and as a volunteer performs the same or similar work as he/she does as an employee.

CHAPTER 19

How to Prepare for Staff Reductions

Until 1984, health care cost increases consistently exceeded those of the Consumer Price Index by a wide variance. The Medicare prospective pricing system that went into effect in October 1983, and the gradual enactment of health care finance and cost containment legislation in many states, drew attention to the need for controlling costs in health care institutions. Under the Medicare prospective pricing law enacted as part of the Social Security Amendments of 1983, the financial incentives for health care institutions changed significantly. Clearly, emphasis was put on cost containment. The Medicare legislation gave health care facilities, for the first time, a financial incentive to keep costs below the established prices. In essence, the prospective pricing plan pays for services rendered to Medicare enrollees as inpatients, on the basis of pre-established "average" prices for diagnosis-related groups (DRGs).

Prospective pricing means that health care facilities need to manage costs within prospectively set revenue limits. The financial incentive for facilities to hold costs under the average set for a given DRG is that they are able to retain the dollar difference. On the other hand, differences between the DRG payment and the facilities' actual costs could spell a loss for the institution. Facilities need to manage costs within the limits of available revenues they receive from the DRG payment system.

Efficient and effective use of a health care facility's human resources are critical to the short-term and long-term viability of health care institutions. Even the best-run health care facility with the most efficient and sensitive management will, in these cost-conscious and competitive times, be forced to lay off employees. Managing under the Medicare prospective pricing system, and in some states, mandated health care cost controls, may require institution-wide changes that will affect the number of health care workers needed. The challenge facing health care chief executive officers is centering on how to remain economically sound while maintaining high quality patient care.

IN THE NEW SCHEME

With DRGs, a facility is paid the same amount regardless of its costs. Thus it can save and even make money if it reduces operating expenses. This new incentive has prompted some institutions to reduce their workforces, particularly since most facilities also have been experiencing a sharp decline in inpatient days.

In general, inpatient stays started to decline with the passage of the 1983 Medicare prospective pricing system. There are a number of explanations for the drop in patient days. Among them:

- Physicians are hospitalizing patients less frequently and sending them home sooner.

- Business, which has been absorbing high health insurance premiums, has been changing health insurance coverage so that employees have an incentive to use the hospital less. Companies are raising deductibles and copayments, and covering treatment in less expensive outpatient settings in full.

- High unemployment in some areas of the country means that many people have lost their health insurance. These people are reluctant to use the hospital for anything but emergency care.

- Hospitals and health care entrepreneurs have been building outpatient centers for "same-day surgery" and other outpatient treatments. These facilities siphon off patients that would previously have been admitted to the hospital as inpatients.

According to one recent study published in the *Harvard Business Review,* "Experts in the field estimate that the U.S. hospital industry has at least 25% too many beds. There are about 1.3 million beds today, but 1.0 to 1.1 million would be sufficient. Even in areas of fast population growth, like the southwestern United States, the need for hospital beds is much less than it was in 1980. Other segments of the health care industry are also suffering from excess capacity. In many large metropolitan areas (San Diego, Portland, and Boston, for example), large physician surpluses exist. Most forecasts predict a large (70,000 or more) nationwide physician surplus by 1990."[1]

LAYOFFS ARE UNPALATABLE

Layoffs are particularly unpalatable for rural hospitals, which are often the single largest employer in town and have been for years operating marginally, both medically and financially.

To preclude layoffs, many administrators have lectured their staffs about cost consciousness and urged doctors to reduce patient tests or have them done outside the facility, where the old reimbursement standards are still applicable. They are also imploring doctors to think twice before admitting patients and to be quicker about discharging them, all of which results in reduced work week hours for employees. In the final analysis, however, health care facilities will need to continually work toward a stable economic vantage point. After testing several alternatives, many will have to conclude that they must cut payroll expenses in order to have a lasting economic base.

Layoffs must be conducted in a humane, though realistic, manner. The facility must retain sufficient staff to provide quality patient care. If this does not happen, employee morale and the institution's standing in the community will suffer.

"Some hospital failures are inevitable," the aforementioned study says. "But it is not in the public interest to have large numbers of hospitals operating in a weakened financial condition, fighting to survive. Strategies for survival are available, and many institutions will, no doubt, respond successfully to the changing health care environment by implementing one or more of these strategies."[1]

HOW TO PREPARE FOR STAFF REDUCTIONS

Terminations require thoughtful and careful planning. They cannot be initiated or implemented overnight or on the spur of the moment. Job security is important to the employees and their families. A decision to reduce staff is a difficult one and should be made only after exhausting all possible alternative solutions. If, however, the decision is made to reduce staff, it is important to remember that such a reduction be made as fairly as possible. As one management study advises, "Employees affected by staff reduction should be given every opportunity to fill other vacant positions for which they may be qualified by experience, education, and/or training."[2]

Staff reduction can be a reduction in force (RIF) or a layoff. A RIF refers to permanent termination of employment resulting from changes in staffing requirements to provide the existing level of health care services. A layoff refers to a temporary situation in which an employee is not working or receiving regular pay but anticipates being recalled as soon as conditions permit. A person on layoff typically is considered an employee for purposes of seniority and union representation.

GENERAL CONSIDERATIONS

Before implementing a staff reduction plan, management should be able to respond effectively to the following questions:

1. What documentation is available to support the need for a staff reduction?

* Decrease in length of stay

- Decrease in utilization (census)

- Poor financial outlook (short-term, long-term)

- Change in services or organizational structure

- Poor productivity (overstaffing).

- It is the responsibility of management not only to gather data that justify the staff reduction but to interpret the appropriate data so that affected parties clearly understand the need for the reduction.

2. Has the facility's general administrative cost of a layoff been determined?

- Potential unemployment claims

- Termination pay (severance, unused time off)

- Benefits (life and medical insurance)

- Liquidation of investment plans

- Early retirement benefits

- Statutorily required payments.

According to an American Hospital Association technical advisory bulletin,

Management should review various alternatives before proceeding with a staff reduction such as appointing a special cost reduction committee to study and recommend solutions, form department task forces to make cost saving suggestions, ask for departmental budget reductions, and solicit recommendations from staff. Prior to the implementation of a staff reduction, an adequate and expeditious review procedure may lend credibility to the process by facilitating recommendations from middle management, unions, and other interested groups that might want to raise concerns for consideration and resolution. The review procedure should be handled by the person or committee responsible for final decisions on staff reductions.[3]

DEALING WITH THE FEARS

Management, after a reduction in force or layoff, must deal with the fears of the remaining staff. The remaining staff can be categorized into two groups:

- Administrative/management

- Operational/clinical

Each has a different perspective in that operational/clinical staff view the administrative and/or management RIF as long overdue and contend that those areas have been top heavy for too long. Wherein the administrative and/or management view RIFs in the operational/clinical areas, particularly in nursing, as valid areas to reduce since the lack of volume/service/census has a direct bearing on those jobs, wherein volume/service/census decreases have no direct impact on the administrative/management personnel. The fear aspects are identical except that group B thinks that group A will be given preferential treatment should the economic picture decline again. Both groups have to be dealt with candidly and openly. Open communication is strongly encouraged. The groups need to know how things are going, the financial picture, plans for the future, and new programs.

RUNNING THE FACILITY: LIFE GOES ON

Life is not the same after a reduction in force or a layoff. Administrative/management personnel need to be much more sensitive to the anxiety prevailing with the operational/clinical personnel. Past practices such as educational trips, expenses, purchases, and paid time off need to be completely thought out. The operational/clinical personnel will develop an acute awareness for what management is up to, and they will display an acute interest in all administrative matters.

PLANNING FOR THE FUTURE

Institutions should develop their RIF policy ahead of time. In the development process it is recommended that the words ''for economic reasons'' not be used as the reason for a reduction or layoff. There may be times when a reduction in force will not be for economic reasons, and management should not lock themselves in at the outset. Give seniority very high consideration when developing a RIF and/or a layoff policy. Don't use RIF or layoff procedures to get rid of marginal performers. That will only attest to the fact that the institution has lived with poor supervision through the years. RIF should not be a substitute for a good discipline process and good supervision.

REACTING TO THE PRESSURE TO REHIRE STAFF

There will be requests from department heads to rehire or recall staff. Those decisions need to be made very carefully. Management will need to closely monitor month-to-month finances, initiate a system of department financial and production reporting and above all else avoid getting sold "a bill of goods," i.e., "those who were not RIF'd or laid off are working harder and therefore deserve help."

LEGAL IMPLICATIONS IN THE RIF OR LAYOFF PROCESS THAT NEED CONSIDERATION

- There could be problems with employment discrimination, such as disparate impact, unequal pay, or age discrimination. For example, combining jobs or reallocating job duties could create equal pay problems.

- Check contracts for bargaining obligations in unionized facilities.

- There may be charges of unfairness by employees on medical leave targeted for layoff.

- Check for conformity with state statutes on final payment of wages and accumulated vacations, and check whether the state has mandated obligations for employers closing all or part of their operations.

ALTERNATIVES TO RIF OR LAYOFFS

Early retirement, freeze on hiring, voluntary resignations, transfers, unpaid leaves of absences, work sharing, and reduced hours of work are some alternatives that can be explored as ways to reduce payroll costs without dramatically altering the institution's labor force. Listed below are some additional alternatives that could result in substantial dollar savings.

- Analyze jobs for common elements and condense jobs where appropriate into fewer levels and distinctions

- Cross-train personnel to handle various job duties in multiple areas

- Avoid duplication of jobs

- Reclassify certain full-time positions to part-time

- Reduce or redeploy certain positions where appropriate within the facility

- Analyze what can be decentralized versus what is more economical to be centralized and thus serve multiple functions or multiple areas

- Look at job-sharing possibilities

- Move from general pay increases to some form of performance-based program

- Abolish automatic step systems

- Analyze career ladders to determine if there are *real differences* in job content and contribution to the organization (such as clerk, senior clerk II, clerk I)

- Review all policies and practices related to overtime

- Review and approve all overtime, permitting no casual overtime

- Analyze all benefit programs and eliminate those that are too costly

- Analyze part-time employee benefit coverages

- Sponsor more employee-subsidized benefit programs

- Monitor shift differentials and consider reducing payment amounts

- Stretch out increases, where appropriate, to sixteen months instead of yearly

- Decrease or defer promotional increases

- Create a labor pool that can be utilized as occupancy rates fluctuate

- Staff for basic level of care, and add and subtract as need dictates

- Analyze current nonexempt workforce and reclassify to exempt status where position meets Fair Labor Standard test for exempt status

- Develop a staffing/position allocation system tied to productivity

- Pay for real performance instead of automatic "follow the leader" market adjustments

- Avoid credential-based pay on "paper mill" credentials frequently unrelated to work done

- Don't ignore pay-range maximums.

Among American industries, the health care industry is still dear to virtually everyone's heart. In our zest to pursue efficiency, to respond to the changing needs of the American public, and to keep up with new health care markets and technology, we must remember that people will continue to look to the health care industry when they are concerned about their own health and when they need medical assistance for their loved ones. We must maintain our image and the public trust. We also need to pursue excellence and efficiency as we move into a new era of health care delivery.

ENDNOTES

1. Dean C. Coddington, Lowell E. Palmquist, and William V. Trollinger, "Strategies for Survival in the Hospital Industry," *Harvard Business Review* (May/June 1985).

2. Hospital Strategies for Staff Reductions, (Kansas City: Management Services Associates, 1984).

3. *Technical Advisory Bulletin--Staff Reductions* (Chicago: American Hospital Association, 1984).

CHAPTER 20

New Horizons and Environments for the Health Care Industry

The United States of America spent over 35 years expanding its health care system. The expansion started right after World War II and developed into an aggregation of varied health care activities. We expanded health manpower and technology. We expanded medical schools, allied health, and nursing personnel technology. As we expanded the U.S. health care system, we also continually expanded the costs. During the growth years, hospital utilization also increased significantly. Access and quality of care were, more or less, the bywords that drove and motivated our health care system. Medicare and Medicaid legislation was enacted in the middle 1960s, based primarily on the theory that some Americans lacked the financial resources to get medical care, and that if someone furnished the cash, then the American public would get all the care they needed. The aggregation of varied health care activities within the conventional U.S. hospital, the freestanding acute care setting, brought together a multitude of health care workers in the American health care system. Up until 1981 most U.S. hospitals were small freestanding institutions.

Starting in 1982, the American health care system profile began changing. The number of proprietary hospitals in the United States rose 14% from 1981 to 1982, according to the American Medical Association's Socioeconomic Monitoring System. The group expects 20 percent of U.S. hospitals to be proprietary by 1990. This does not mean that for-profits were the only growing hospitals during that period. In some areas of the country, nonprofit hospital groups now rival for-profit hospitals in numbers and size of institutions. For example, the New York City Health & Hospital Corporation has more than 8,000 beds. The American health care system is undergoing metamorphosis.

Hospitals are broadening their efforts to market health care by running not just acute care hospitals, but also psychiatric programs, ambulatory outpatient centers, drug and alcohol detoxification centers, home health care programs, rehabilitation centers, commercial laboratories, health maintenance organizations, adult day care centers, diagnostic centers, and congregate housing programs.

THE BATTLE FOR CONTROL OF THE HEALTH CARE MARKET

In the battle for control of the health care market, for-profit facilities are accused of--as articulated by Dr. Arnold Relman in a debate on the issue--"jeopardizing education and research and rising rather than lowering costs to the consumers. It is also advocated that for-profits create a crisis in values with their conflicting responsibilities to shareholders and community members.''[1] The profit chains' access to capital is cited as an unfair advantage in the struggle for the health care market. There are several questions remaining to be answered before a final chapter can be written on the subject:

- ''Is health care a commodity like food, fuel, or housing--and subject to the free market--or is it essentially different, to be run by Main Street rather than Wall Street?'' Dr. Relman asked.[1]

- In the struggle for market share, little is said or written about the health care worker.

  - What are the implications for management, employees, and the unions? Will there be more or less unionization?

  - Will management need a more decentralized approach as health care facilities branch out?

One author suggests that

''The health care complex is subject to such strong forces of change
from so many directions that health care managers must maintain an
active awareness of the important facts, data, and emerging trends in
various components and sectors of the health care system. Only in
this manner can they discharge their duties toward, and play an active
role in, the formulation of those health policies relating various issues
surrounding the organization, management, financing, and delivery of
health care.''[2]

There is a trend developing wherein freestanding hospitals are looking to be associated with a ''system.'' If the trend continues, by 1986 nearly half of the nation's hospitals will be part of a multi-institutional system. Multihospital systems, one of the fastest growing segments in the health care delivery industry, have become a powerful force in the health care field. The range of systems goes all the way from a two-hospital system to the real giants such as the Hospital Corporation of America, which either owns or manages nearly 400 institutions. The Center for Multi-institutional Arrangements of the American Hospital Association has more than 250 systems on its rosters.

There are varied opinions as to the reasons for the growth and popularity of multisystems. Some of the reasons given most frequently are: it makes the hospital more efficient, there are savings to be realized in the purchasing of goods, more administrative services become available, capital acquisition become easier, and a multitude of other economics.

Also, being part of a large system helps to attract a higher level of professional management to the institution. The health care industry of the future will need health care executives with vision who welcome rather than are afraid of change, who are not afraid to ask hard questions and most importantly make hard decisions and take risks. If the chief executive officer cannot answer honestly questions related to the future survival of the institution, then he/she should consider a change in professional employment.

NEW HORIZONS

Health industry employment skyrocketed in the 1970s and, although it slowed in the early 1980s, is expected to outpace employment in other business sectors through 1995, according to a study by the AFL-CIO. Hospital employment alone rose 51 percent between 1971 and 1983 and, because of projected demand increases from a growing elderly population and advances in medical technology, is expected to surpass overall U.S. employment growth, rising 39 percent between 1983 and 1995, the report says.[3]

However, hospitals' share of health industry employment is declining, according to the AFL-CIO report, which drew on data from federal and state agencies and the health care industry. In 1972, hospitals employed 60 percent of all health care workers, but by 1982 that percentage had dropped to 55 percent. The report shows that employment expansion rates for the hospital segment of the health care industry rose 31 percent between 1970 and 1976, 22 percent between 1976 and 1982, and had virtually no increase between 1982 and 1983. Meanwhile, employment in other health care segments rose 61 percent between 1970 and 1976, 37 percent between 1976 and 1982, and 3 percent between 1982 and 1983.[3]

The fastest growing segments of health industry employment were convalescent institutions and a category labeled "other," which included all health services not classified as hospitals, convalescent institutions, physicians' offices, or dentists' offices. Convalescent facilities' employment grew 127 percent between 1971 and 1983, employing 1.3 million workers in 1983. Services labeled "other," which included outpatient clinics, freestanding emergency centers, HMOs and other health service providers, grew 126 percent between 1971 and 1983, employing 944,000 workers in 1983.[3] (See Table 20-1).

NEW ENVIRONMENTS

Health care employees, who may or may not have survived an economic reduction in force or a layoff, are finding themselves in new work environments

Table 20-1   Workers in the Health Services Industry by Segment (in thousands)[3]

Year	Hospitals	Total (excluding hospitals)	Convalescent institutions	Physicians' offices	Dentists' offices	Other
1971	2,878	1,727	590	486	234	418
1972	2,914	1,936	651	557	255	473
1976	3,568	2,572	933	657	332	650
1980	3,947	3,280	1,185	756	407	933
1982	4,341	3,518	1,217	898	415	988
1983	4,348	3,615	1,342	888	441	944
Percentage change: 1971 to 1983						
	51%	109%	127%	85%	88%	126%

as a result of hospitals seeking to market health care differently. These new work environments, not necessarily located within a traditional hospital building, include:

- Home Care Programs

- Rehabilitation Centers

- Ambulatory Outpatient Centers

- Health Maintenance Organizations

- Adult Day Care Centers

- Commercial Laboratories

- Alcohol/Drug Detoxification Centers

- Psychiatric Programs

- Congregate Housing Programs

- Diagnostic Centers.

The history of labor relation issues for these satellite center employees has yet to be lived and recorded. One major question has, to date, come to the surface: Does management need to deal with satellite center employees differently?

The answer is yes! They do need to be treated or dealt with differently, because they feel as if they are out of step with some of their peers who are still working in the traditional hospital setting and are not "in on things."

In the final analysis management needs to design its human resource programs to address the following for its satellite employees:

- Recognize their work.

- Make them feel as if they are still part of the hospital.

- Be sympathetic and help them with personal problems.

- Communicate job security to them.

- Give them wages and benefits comparable to hospital employees'.

- Give them plenty of opportunity to expand their job knowledge through in-service and educational opportunities.

- Give them promotion opportunities comparable to hospital employees'.

- Show your loyalty toward them.

- Give them good working conditions.

- Be fair and tactful in your discipline process.

Most people enter the health care profession because they care about people and their needs. IBM, while not a health care provider, has a relevant three-point company philosophy that states in part:

- respect the individual employee and those you service

- provide the best service as an employee or as an organization

- excel in what you do as an employee or as an organization.

The IBM philosophy deliberately does not directly address cost, efficiency, profit, or technology. The assumption is that if one does the three listed things correctly, the balance will fall into place.

It would behoove the health care industry as it moves into new horizons to consider adopting a basic philosophy that embraces *respect, service, and excellence.*

ENDNOTES

1. "The Great Debate" held April 3, 1985, at the New England Hospital Assembly, Boston. Arnold Relman, M.D., editor of the *New England Journal of Medicine*, spoke as a critic of the for-profit approach. Thomas Frist, Jr., President and CEO of Hospital Corporation of America (HCA), Nashville, Tenn., spoke in favor of the for-profit approach. Ben Jacques was special correspondent for the American Hospital Association, Chicago.

2. Samuel Levey and N. Paul Loomba, *Health Care Administration: A Management Perspective.* 1983: J.B. Lippincott Co.

3. E. Sekscenski. *The Health Services Industry in the United States.* American Federation of Labor and Congress of Industrial Organizations, August, 1984.

CASE STUDY

A FOUR-WEEK CAMPAIGN TO DETER A UNIONIZATION ATTEMPT

Note: This is a hypothetical case study of a unionization effort that was triggered because of a staff reduction at Express Care, Inc. The only issue in the campaign was job security.

Background: Express Care, Inc., a division of the XYZ Medical Center, had a long-standing employee relations policy that advocated that, since management adhered to a philosophy of continued fair employee relations practices, there was no need for any third party(ies) to intervene between the employees and the management of Express Care, Inc.

The Express Care, Inc. employee relations policy stressed, among other things, that the facility would do all that was reasonably possible to meet the needs of their total staff and to foster and to promulgate "competitive wage/salary programs, competitive benefits programs, steady employment, and career mobility."

The organization had not experienced previous union activity and had enjoyed relatively good employee/employer relations.

Express Care, Inc. had 20 first-line supervisors who were responsible for the day-to-day supervision of employees. Except for some minor grievances related to supervisors assigning undesirable shift work to employees with no regard for seniority, the institution experienced little labor turmoil. Grievances were always resolved quickly and fairly. Most grievance decisions were in favor of employees.

Channels of communication were always kept open. The institution used bulletin boards, departmental meetings, shift meetings and had a widely circulated in-house publication called "What's Happening."

The most frequent employee complaints were directed towards administration. Employees frequently commented that administration was "top-heavy"--"too many chiefs and not enough Indians." The CEO overlooked the comments and considered them "typical complaints from operating departments." There also existed a tendency on the part of the CEO to accommodate the medical staff on all issues and at all cost to "keep peace in the family."

A reduction in force became necessary in January 1985 as a result of the federal prospective pricing system (PPS) that went into effect in October 1983, wherein hospitals are reimbursed under Medicare based on a fixed price (rate per discharge) for 468 different categories of illness, called diagnosis related groups (DRGs). In order to reduce its labor cost and bring them into line with current and anticipated revenues, management determined it would have to terminate 20 employees from housekeeping, dietary, maintenance, and clerical areas.

Express Care, Inc. used the following criteria to determine who would be terminated:

- The personnel department was asked to prepare a list of approximately 20 positions to be eliminated. The personnel department felt uniquely qualified for this task since it had been living with a ''restricted hiring'' procedure for the past several months and knew which departments had complied with the spirit of the restricted hiring procedure and which had not.

- The instruction given to personnel from the CEO was that no clinical areas would be involved in the reduction.

- The personnel department prepared the list of 20 positions and, in most cases, used seniority as the final deciding factor. Three of those selected for termination were not the least senior employees in their job classification.

- It was decided that the terminations would be effective immediately and the employees would be paid for time in lieu of notice but would not work beyond the date of notification.

- Final paychecks, termination notices, and state unemployment compensation procedures were prepared for those to be terminated.

- The CEO asked the respective department heads to meet alone with the employees and explain the reasons to them.

- The effective date of the termination was on a Monday so that those terminated could begin to look for other work immediately instead of worrying all weekend over something they could not immediately do something about.

- Rumors just before the terminations were rampant and, to management's surprise, several troublesome employees volunteered to be terminated, and management gladly accommodated them.

Those effected by the reduction in force were given assistance in finding other employment. Only five out of the 20 involved in the reduction were placed in other non-health care industries within the community.

In March 1985 a group of employees, mostly from the departments in which the reductions had taken place, contacted two local trade unions. One of the unions agreed to initiate action for a collective bargaining contract with Express Care, Inc.

Within two weeks after the union organizer appeared on the scene, the CEO received a recognition demand letter in which the union stated that it represented the majority of employees in the clerical and service areas. The union asked for recognition as the bargaining agent for these units. The CEO declined to recognize the union in the basis of the recognition demand letter and referred the union to the National Labor Relations Board to file a petition.

A hearing was scheduled by the NLRB within 30 days after the referral. Two units were found appropriate (clerical and service), and an election date was scheduled. The vice-president--human resources, the CEO, and the attorney for Express Care, Inc. designed a four-week campaign to counter the unionization attempt. The campaign was designed to start specifically four weeks before the election date. No actions were to take place before the start of the designed program.

What follows are the Express Care, Inc. literature and guidelines. The material can be modified to fit any size health care facility and to respond to any issue(s) that may have caused a unionization attempt.

SELECTED READING

Bean, Joseph J. Jr., and Rene Laliberty. *Understanding Hospital Labor Relations.* Reading, MA: Addison-Wesley Publishing Co., 1977.

Chaney, Warren H., and Thomas R. Beech. *The Union Epidemic.* Rockville: Aspen Systems Corp., 1976.

Laliberty, Rene, and Joseph J. Bean, Jr., *Decentralizing Hospital Management.* Reading, MA: Addison-Wesley Publishing Co., 1980.

Metzger, Norman, and Joseph M. Ferentino. *The Arbitration and Grievance Process--A Guide for Health Care Supervisors.* Rockville, MD: Aspen Systems Corp., 1983.

Metzger, Norman; Ferentino, Joseph M.; and Kurger, K. *When Health Care Employees Strike.* Rockville, MD: Aspen Systems Corp., 1984.

Metzger, Norman, and Dennis D. Pointer. *Labor-Management Relations in the Health Services Industry--Theory and Practice.* Volume 4, *Sourcebook series.* Washington: Science & Health Publications, 1972.

USE OF CASE STUDY

This hypothetical case study provides the reader with a useful medium for testing and applying some of the principles, ideas, and policies in this textbook. It is an opportunity for some of the material to be considered for practical applications within a health care facility, and it is also an opportunity for managers to use the book in educational discussion sessions with their supervisory staff members.

DISCUSSION TOPICS

- **When the employees seek the union.** When it is the employees who initiate the union aggression, management has often had many opportunities in the past to identify that there is unrest, unhappiness, or a general pattern of dissatisfaction around specific issues. It is vital that members of the administrative and management staff attempt to identify

as specifically as possible all primary issues and then all
secondary or contributing issues.

- **When the union organizer seeks membership.** When it
is the union or the professional association functioning as a
union that attempts to seek membership and to organize the
nonunion employees for purposes of representation to seek
collective bargaining, the success of the organizer depends
largely on his ability to identify those issues--wages, benefits, hours, and general working conditions--around which
employees find various degrees of dissatisfaction. Many
employees will openly express their concerns, problems,
and insecurities to the union organizer at union meetings or
in impromptu conferences. Many employees, however, do
not want to become involved and maintain a closed mouth
along with a closed mind insofar as union membership is
concerned.
    As hard as it is for the union organizer to ascertain spe-
cific issues, it may be equally hard for management to
identify such issues. There is, in a sense, a race between
management and the union organizer to determine who can
identify the issues in the most clear and specific manner
and propose a remedy for such issues in such a way as to
gain the support of the employee.
    The union organizer will always assume that manage-
ment, in daily contact with the employees, will be apprised
of the issues. Those in management realize that this is not
always the case.
    The union organizer has an additional advantage in that
by failing to identify the real issues, he or she can often
create suggested or reflected issues to the employees based
on the experience of the organizer in other campaigns.
There are normal patterns of employee concerns over security of job, of wage, and of a future, that can be used as bait
to open discussions with the employee and eventually
identify the real problems.
    It is important to keep in mind that management has es-
tablished a track record, whereas the union needs to establish such a record to gain employee confidence. If the employees have been satisfied with what management has
done in the past, they are likely to maintain that degree of
satisfaction as management responds to current and future

problems. On the other hand, employees know what the
union has done through other collective bargaining agreements to assist in meeting employee needs elsewhere. This
union track record is often used as part of the organizing
strategy, with the organizers displaying collective bargaining agreements, arbitration awards, and other evidence of
their achievements and effectiveness. To oversimplify the
situation, it can be stated that the party that can demonstrate
to the employees the ability to provide realistic security and
justify the employees' confidence will eventually gain the
employees' support.

It is the intent of this case study campaign strategy plan to
assist management in being the victor in this competitive
role.

CHAPTER APPLICATION TO DISCUSSION TOPICS

Chapter 3   Positive Supervisory Practices to Maintain Nonunion
Status in a Health Care Facility

Chapter 7   The Union: Friend or Foe to Management?

Chapter 8   Basic Components of the Union Election Process:
Bargaining Units and Decertification

Chapter 16   The Role of Participative Management in Employee
Relations

Chapter 17   Understanding Morale Survey Data

Chapter 19   How to Prepare for Staff Reductions

Chapter 20   New Horizons and New Environments for the Health
Care Industry

STUDY GUIDES

It is suggested that the case group leader assign different
chapters as required reading to various members of the study group.
Members should then be prepared to discuss with the group the

content of their chapter and its applicability to the case study topics. This study process can be repeated and different chapters of the book assigned to members of the group making various assumptions, such as:

- Express Care, Inc. lost the election--why?

- Express Care, Inc. won the election--why?

- How could staff reductions have been handled better?

- If Express Care, Inc. needs to have another staff reduction, how should it be communicated?

- How could the CEO have precluded the perception employees had that administration was "proprofessional"?

- How could the four-week campaign strategy have been improved?

- Was the four-week campaign offensive to the reader? If so, why?

EXPRESS CARE, INC., DIVISION OF XYZ MEDICAL CENTER

Strategy of a Four-Week Union Campaign

During a union campaign, because the stakes are often irreversible, no important communication can be left to chance. It is the matter of stating clearly the position management wants understood and accepted, and reenforcing from as many points of view as possible the flow of that information to the employees. Each week of the campaign, therefore, we will concentrate on a separate theme. A concentration of letters, bulletins, handouts, posters, and conferences will center around a single topic on the premise that what one employee hears the other misses, and the one that missed receiving the communication may in turn pick it up through a second, third, or fourth alternative means of communication.

The backbone of employee-management relationships is the established relationship between the employee and the immediate first-line supervisor. All representatives of higher levels of management merely represent a force intended to assist the supervisor and the employees get the job done. The intent of our campaign is to establish in the minds of the employees a sense of realistic security, realistic confidence in management, and harmonious relationships.

The following campaign material must be studied carefully and understood by the governing board and the administrative team before the vital function of supervisory action commences. The stakes are high. The reluctant supervisor, the unwilling supervisor, and the dissident supervisor all constitute threats to management's "nonunion" position. Where there is confidence in the capacity of the supervisor to function adequately in support of management's position, such a supervisor will be given every opportunity to seek guidance, counsel, or help and given every kind of instruction, guidance, or direction possible. The supervisor who raises more questions than confidence, however, will need close supervision and may actually require the presence and ongoing support of the department head or higher administrative staff to be assured that the positions taken by management are adhered to and that the anticipated program is actually implemented as planned.

Constant surveillance or monitoring of the campaign is essential. Continuous and adequate documentation of both positive and negative behavioral patterns by both management team members and employees is equally vital. The results of management's interest and efforts will be counted in the ballot box.

/s/ _____
Chief Executive Officer
Express Care, Inc.

Details of Basic Campaign Strategy

Observing the specific strategy objectives set forth for our campaign prior to the union election, the following strategy has been agreed upon:

I.   The weekly campaign approach

    A. We will define the specific objectives for the week's campaign by identifying one critical issue and its related issues and designing the total campaign around these issues to meet a specific set of objectives.

B. We will use a multifaceted approach in order to reach the employees from several directions and to reinforce what has already been communicated by some other means.

C. On a weekly basis three, four, or five different approaches will be used as follows:

   1. A short personal letter from the Chief Executive Officer.

   2. A bulletin board poster that can be widely posted throughout the facility.

   3. A specific set of guidelines for supervisors for the purpose of conducting small group conferences or informal conversations with two or more employees.

   4. A handout for supervisors that will restate and reinforce the content of the supervisor's conferences or conversations.

   5. A paycheck insert that will focus attention on a few, very specific issues and reinforce and/or recap all previous efforts.

D. We will conduct mixed small group meetings, 30 minutes in length or less, with the Chief Executive Officer to present briefly some position important to the campaign and to respond to employee questions. Such meetings will be carefully planned, an outline prepared in advance, and a tape recording of the session made to protect the facility against charges of unfair labor practices.

E. We will develop a simple motto, slogan, or logo that can be attached to all campaign material and become a symbol of the facility's position. In the final days of the campaign, it can simply be used as a quick reminder of all that has been said in the past. This will be something short and simple such as--

1. THINK ABOUT IT.

2. BECAUSE WE CARE.

3. LET'S GET ORGANIZED--NOT UNIONIZED.

4. WE NEED UNITY, NOT A UNION.

F. All supervisors will report, record, document, summarize, and evaluate every aspect of the campaign to determine strengths, weaknesses, trends, and alternate approaches.

/s/ _____
Vice-President--Human Resources

Guide for Supervisors: Week 1

Objective: It is intended that the first week campaign clarify for the employees the details of their legal rights, the significance of signing a union card and making the union representative an agent, and the process and details of the NLRB conducted election.

Supervisory Support: The ultimate strengths and effectiveness of the campaign will be determined by the relationship between the immediate supervisors and the employees involved. Conversations between the supervisors and the employees will be most important. The supervisors will be supported through a briefing session concerning the topics of the week. A letter will be sent to concerned employees from the Chief Executive Officer. Bulletins will be prepared for bulletin board posting. A handout will be prepared for distribution to the employees by the supervisors. The following supervisor's guide is intended to assist the supervisors in the relationship with the employee. The handout for the employee is intended to provide supervisors with an excuse to make contact. Copies of all printed materials will be made available.

Communication Guideline: The following topics should be discussed by the supervisors with concerned employees--preferably an open, informal discussion involving not more than two or three employees at a time.

1. When the NLRB election has been set, the facility will be obligated to post official notice. The supervisor should stress the date, the time, and the place. Review the description of the bargaining unit and identify who in the department may vote and who may not vote.

2. Indicate that all eligible employees should vote. The vote will be on secret ballot. Indicate that an employee who has signed a union card can still vote "No." Neither management nor the union will know how anyone votes. (See Exhibit 1).

3. If no union authorization card has been signed, indicate to the employee that caution should be exercised before signing such a card. Stress that signing a union card makes the union the agent for the employee. The union becomes the sole representative of the employee. The employee can no longer represent himself directly with management.

4. If an employee wants not to be involved but is included in the bargaining unit, stress the importance of a "No" vote by this employee. The employee may lose his right if the union should win the election and the employee does not want to join the union, does not want to pay union dues, does not want to attend union meetings and does not want to be limited to the conditions of a negotiated collective bargaining agreement. The outcome of the election will determine if the facility is to be unionized or to remain nonunion. The outcome will be determined by the number of votes cast and not the number eligible to vote. If one more than one-half of the votes cast are for the union (a "Yes" vote), the union will represent all employees. To remain uninvolved and to maintain a nonunion status, the employee must vote "No."

5. The employee rights are important. Employees have the right to join or to refuse to join the union. They have the rights to sign a union card or to refuse to sign a union card, refuse to talk with union organizers, refuse to permit union organizers in their homes, refuse to take telephone calls from union agents, and refuse to discuss the matter with fellow employees.

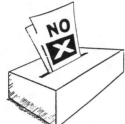

EVEN IF YOU
HAVE SIGNED A
UNION CARD OR
HAVE BEEN A
UNION MEMBER

YOU ARE 100% NO
FREE TO VOTE

FOR NO DUES
FOR NO STRIKES *Vote* NO UNION
FOR NO UNION RULES

Exhibit 1

6. The law requires that a list of the names and addresses of employees designated in the bargaining unit be sent to the NLRB in duplicate so that a copy can be sent to the union. The facility resents having to do this but is obligated by law. Indicate to the employees that this will give the union an opportunity to put pressure on those employees who have not yet signed union cards.

7. Stress that the facility believes that it is in the employee's own best interest to vote "No" in the election. Specific information will be given to the employee to support this position in the next several weeks. The employee will be subject to union propaganda and should carefully study such propaganda before responding to it. The facility will hold small group meetings with employees to explain hospital information and to react to union information.

Handouts: The supervisor will be provided with a handout on specific questions and direct answers to be given to the employee after discussions.

Record and Report: It is important to maintain the one-on-one list of "Yes," "Uncertain," and "No" votes so that at any point there is an updated list available by which to ascertain strengths or weaknesses. The supervisor is asked to maintain a notebook to record everything that might be significant with regard to the union campaign, including interviews with particular reactions or results, any information learned about union meetings, union literature, and union interviews. Beware of rumors, and report any to the Vice-President--Human Resources.

Specific Questions and Answers

The management of this facility would like to give you honest and straightforward answers to a number of questions that have been raised in connection with the election to be held soon:

Question: If I signed a union authorization card, must I vote for the union?

Answer: Absolutely not. The election is secret. You can vote anyway you want.

Question: Is there any way that the union, the hospital, or the NLRB can know how I vote?

Answer: Absolutely not. Your vote will be in absolute secrecy. You do not sign your ballot. You place it in the ballot box yourself.

Question: If the union loses the election and I am a union supporter, will I lose my job?

Answer: Absolutely not. All employees will be treated alike by Express Care, Inc.

Question: If the union wins the election, will union members be given preferential treatment?

Answer: Absolutely not. All employees will be treated alike by Express Care, Inc.

Question: Will my job be more secure if I vote for the union?

Answer: Absolutely not. The best job security you have is a well-run, efficient facility. We believe the tension, strife, conflict, and possible strikes that could occur with a union at this facility could hurt our image and our efficiency. If the facility is hurt, it would hurt everyone's job security. The recent reduction of 20 jobs at Express Care, Inc. was very unfortunate; however, it was a very necessary move in order to strengthen our financial position during these very difficult times for the health care industry.

Question: If the union called me out on an economic strike to support its negotiating demands, would I be guaranteed that I could return to my job?

Answer: Absolutely not. The facility must maintain its operations in the interest of patient care. The law would give the hospital the right to hire a permanent replacement for you.

Question: Are there any advantages to me to joining and belonging to the union?

Answer: Absolutely not, insofar as your employment at this facility. We pay your wages and provide your benefits--not the union. The record of wage increases and benefit improvements is obvious. This was done without your need to pay union dues, to attend union meetings, or to assume the risk of demonstrating, picketing, or striking. We have not just made promises--we have delivered. The union can only make promises.

As the election date approaches you can expect to hear many promises from the union of how things will be once Express Care, Inc. is unionized. You can expect to hear many criticisms of what we have done or failed to do even though the union does not have the facts to make such a criticism. You will hear more from us on why we feel it is in your best interest not to have a union and why you should vote "no." This will raise other questions in your mind. We ask that you consult your supervisor for a direct answer.

Important Thoughts about Union Promises

The union has promised improved wages, benefits, and job security (no layoffs, etc.), but each promise is subject to negotiation. The law does not require management to do other than negotiate in good faith.

Management has not merely promised but has delivered. Without payment of dues, initiation fees, or attendance at union meetings you have received . . .

Wage increases each year: We have voluntarily given either a general increase, merit and/or top-of-scale bonus.

New benefits: A recent employer-paid dental plan and two new differentials for weekends and holidays.

Communication: We keep you posted on the progress of all our programs and projects; as a matter of fact, we are the only health care facility that we know of that has a 10-point communication program in effect for our employees.

Job security: Yes, job security! Express Care, Inc. has been in business for 50 years, and the unavoidable reduction in force we had in January 1985 was the first staff reduction we've ever had--that's not a bad record.

Some employees actually believe that what the union promises is what they are entitled to. This leads to anticipation and then disappointment. This creates tension and sometimes hostility. The union promise becomes a demand that may lead to a strike.

Keep in mind that until someone puts something in the pot, no one can take something out. The union produces no products and creates no service that will produce income.

Management must plan for the health care services that the employees produce. Management must sell those services, render a bill, and collect the money to fill the pot so that everyone can get a fair share.

A "yes" vote will not fill the pot. Negotiations cannot deliver what is not there.

A "no" vote will restore harmony to Express Care, Inc. so that management and employees can work cooperatively to produce and provide for the benefit of all.

THIS IS SOMETHING FOR YOU TO THINK ABOUT!

Guide for Supervisors: Week 2

Objective: It is the intention of the second week's campaign to promote understanding among the supervisory staff as to why we must oppose unionization of our workforce by looking at both the impact of the unionization on management and the problem from the employee point of view. It is vital to offset union propaganda that management's opposition to the union's organizing effort suggests management has something to gain at the employee's expense if the union effort can be defeated. It must be pointed out that the employee has something to lose through unionization also. The theme "Unity, Not Union" should be stressed and repeated every way possible. The facility's track record of wage improvements, benefit improvements, and job security should be stated and restated, emphasizing that all of this was accomplished without negotiation and without the employee sharing some of the benefits by paying dues to a union.

Supervisory Support: Continue to build the one-on-one relationship with the employee. The supervisors must have a briefing session early the second week to review all problems and progress resulting from the effort of the first week and to receive this guideline and other materials for the second week campaign. The continued emphasis of the personal relationship between the supervisor and the employee must be maintained. This will be supported with a letter from the Chief Executive Officer to be mailed early and a poster on all bulletin boards dealing with the facility's track record on personnel program improvements. A particular handout on why we oppose unions must be used by the supervisors as an opener for the conversation with employees and as something to leave with them to reinforce the conversation. GOOD LUCK! ASK FOR HELP IF NEEDED.

    Communication Guideline: The following topics must be discussed by the supervisor with concerned employees, preferably in an open, informal discussion--not more than two or three employees at a time.

1. Raise the question with the employees as to whether they think we favor or disfavor the unionization of the workforce and why they think so. Be careful not to ask the employees for their position or his reasons--only their opinion about our position.

2. Point out to the employees that there actually would be some benefits to us if our workforce were to be unionized.

3. Spell out for the employees reasons we oppose unionism from the *employee's* point of view.

4. Point out the benefits the employees have received based on our published track record emphasizing both wages and benefits;--none of which cost time, effort, or money to the employees. Don't be hesitant to mention our 50-year job security track record.

5. Emphasize the value of the benefit package by converting time and cash benefits to a total dollar value.

6. Do not project either specifically or generally further benefit improvements or further wage improvements lest this be construed as a promise.

7. Provide the employees with appropriate handout materials.

8. Use frequently the phrase "We need unity, not a union."

9. In a free, sincere, informal manner invite the employees to consult you on any concerns that they have about what our position might be or how the union propaganda has attempted to counter our position. Take the position that you are attempting to be a friend in this time of confusion and tension. Impress upon the employees that only they will decide whether we will be unified or unionized. Let the employees know that by law management may not question them about their position and feelings on the matter, but by the same law, management can respond to the employees who are willing to discuss the issues and raise questions for the supervisor's response.

Record and Report: It is important to maintain the one-on-one list of "Yes," "Uncertain" and "No" votes so that at any point there is an updated list available by which to ascertain strengths or weaknesses. Supervisors are asked to maintain continuing notes on interviews, conferences, questions, and problems.

Why Express Care, Inc. Opposes Unionism

One might ask, "Why does Express Care, Inc. oppose the union?" Is there something in it for management? Does management want to keep the employees from getting something to which they are entitled?

Actually, we have very little to lose if we have a union, but YOU DO. We would have some advantages:

● Our labor costs would be set by the contract, would be fixed and could be projected for the one-, two- or three-year period of the contract. There would be no interim adjustments and responses to changes in the cost of living and working conditions. With the new DRG reimbursement system for Medicare patients, that would stabilize our labor costs.

● Personnel policies and benefits would be frozen in contract language and would be set without review, revision, or improvement for the duration of the contract. That, too, would be helpful in a changing economic environment.

- We need not apologize to the public for future rate increases--we could simply blame the union for the increased costs.

- The union grievance procedure might surface problems more quickly since the employees might forfeit their right to use the grievance system if filing the complaint was delayed--thus giving management the opportunity to settle problems sooner.

- A labor contract works two ways--for the employees and for the institution--and we might be able to lean on the union to enforce employee discipline.

- And there are others, but . . .

Why does Express Care, Inc. oppose a union if it has these and other benefits? The reasons are simple and clear. They are:

- Why not enjoy all of your wages and benefits? Why share part with the union by paying dues, fees, fines, or assessments? The union contributed nothing to the payment of better wages and improved benefits. We made the effort to make these possible. We want the employees to benefit to the fullest extent. (See Exhibit 2.)

- Who understands the employee relations problems better than you and management? If we know enough and care enough, we can settle our own problems without outside interference and without the expense of lawyers, counselors, or representatives, whose fees could better be used to benefit all of us here.

- Management wants to satisfy the needs of the facility and its workforce. Too often it is learned too late that much of what must be negotiated is necessary to satisfy the union and has no benefit to us and our workforce.

- The inflexibility of wages and benefits as stated in a work contract might in this rapidly changing period of economics

For NO Dues, NO Strikes, NO Picket Lines . . .

VOTE

put your X in box marked

NO ☒

Exhibit 2

become a serious handicap to both retaining and recruiting necessary staff.

- Interference with our primary responsibility--quality patient care--becomes very real when a collective bargaining agreement establishes job jurisdictions or limits technological improvements, development of performance standards, exercise of a good performance evaluation, self-determination of training needs, appropriate application of discipline, and other conditions that make this facility a harmonious place in which to work.

- In the effort to create one team of management working closely with the workforce, it is soon realized that the union creates splinter groups, often competing among each other and always serving as a confrontation force in opposition to what management must do to maintain a healthy and viable health care facility.

- Many professionals and/or health care workers do not want to be subjected to union working conditions despite the belief that there are some benefits to the employees. This handicaps effective hospital recruitment, making it difficult to find good personnel to work side-by-side with you.

- Time might better be spent in improving our image, working closer with the medical staff, making improvements in patient care systems and services, or reviewing the employee relations program, wages, benefits, and policies--instead of responding to union-created problems, concerns, and questions, preparing for negotiations, and preparing for and preparing for arbitration. Just look at the time that has been devoted to this current union campaign that could have better been spent on the continual improvement of the facility. Think of the time you have spent. Time is precious. We need to use it to improve what we are doing and the benefits we derive from our actions.

- There is always the danger of work interruptions, picketing, and strikes and the need to recognize picket lines--all of which places the patients in serious jeopardy. Yet if management must say ''no'' to some union demand, these are the only coercive tactics that the union has in attempting to force management to say "yes." Management does not FORCE but REVIEWS, REVISES, AND IMPROVES its program of services, its program of income and expense control, and its program of personnel benefits and wage improvements. Hard work, not force, makes the improvement possible. We are sorry we had to have a reduction in force, but would it have been better to close our facility rather than make a hard economic decision?

- Too often collective bargaining is for the benefit of the union, and you and we must do what the union wants done. The union will want to involve you in the union welfare programs over which neither you nor the institution will have any control or voice. Our business office will be expected to handle the collection of union dues and make reports to the union. We will be expected to provide the union with lists of new names of employees as well as those terminated. This involves us in union business, which we do not want to be in--our business is health care.

THINK ABOUT IT. We are a nonprofit corporation. Management and the employees are paid a competitive wage. No one benefits from poor working conditions, poor communications and work relationships, or poor wages and benefits. For management to benefit, your role, your relationship, and your reward--the performance and cooperation within this facility--must be improved. A satisfied employee does a better job. A better job improves the image of the facility. A better image brings the interest of the better physician and assures the facility of patients. The patients provide the income from which we must all take our fair share. Unity, not a union, will benefit us all.

What are the Vital Signs for a Healthy Health Care Facility?

The best security an employee can have is a healthy health care facility that functions in harmony, that is compatible within itself, that can provide the job, the job security and the job benefits sought by all.

What are the signs of a healthy health care facility?

- Employees are compatible with the operational philosophy so that management and the employees function as compatible partners sharing the same basic principles or beliefs.

- Employees and management strive to achieve commonly understood and accepted operational goals and objectives.

- We are able to attract and maintain competent employees and the work environment stimulates professional and personal growth and development.

- Employees working with management show vision and imagination and can project this institution into new avenues of health care delivery, providing for those not yet served and expanding into new services. This is called MARKETING--a new venture for health care facilities.

- Employees and management perform interdependently with one another, avoiding the necessity of creating empires, building dynasties, playing politics, or leaning on outside representation to do what can better be done through mutual interaction and support.

- Employees and management can freely communicate one to another to establish an atmosphere of mutual need satisfaction in an atmosphere that promotes constructive criticism as freely as it promotes recognition and praise.

- Management working through cooperative employees strives to properly utilize all of its resources, facilities, tools and apparatus, materials and supplies, attitudes, and talent expressed through the workforce--all in the interest of efficient delivery of health care services to the community.

- There is an environment of mutual trust--management for the employees but, equally important, employees for management. Such an atmosphere emerges when there is openness and honesty. It leads to a sense of personal and professional freedom and eventually a community interest or sense of oneness. Management and employees truly become one force, a team.

- The general environment strives to avoid undue and petty criticism, destructive and hurtful attitudes, and waste and exploitation, and provides instead for the proposal of new ideas, recommendations for improvement and the development of its people, and productive contributions to the pursuit of excellence.

- Both employees and management are effective in doing the right things while maintaining an atmosphere through which each can freely point out the deficiencies or failures of the other without fear of undue criticism or retribution.

- The members of the management staff are viewed by the employees as friends doing their own thing in the interest of all and not as a symbol of authority.

Guide for Supervisors: Week 3

Objective: The intention of this week's campaign is to pose to the employees the actual dangers of unionism in terms of work stoppages, picketing, and strikes that may result from unrealistic union promises or from the type of promises that become campaign issues and therefore, in the event of a union victory, negotiating demands. It is intended that the employees understand specific facts about the involved union, its financial structures, its officers, its loyalty oath, and other conditions that the employees might view negatively if they understood them. It is important to achieve an understanding by the employees of the limited way in which the union gives them support in contrast to the major way they are expected to give support to the union.

Supervisory Supports: It is intended that the supervisor keep maintaining close one-on-one relationships with the employees. In this week of the campaign there should be a letter from the Chief Executive Officer and a series of meetings of mixed groups of employees with a presentation by either the Chief Executive Officer, Vice-President--Human Resources, or labor counsel. The theme of the meeting will be to challenge the union. A handout will be prepared in accordance with the challenge and distributed to the employees to raise doubt in their minds that the union is their source of job security.

Communication Guideline: The formal meeting with mixed groups of employees will be set up for 30 minutes per group with a limit of approximately 15 to 20 employees per group and with provision to tape record the session so as to offset any danger of an unfair labor practice accusation. The presentation will be carefully outlined with a script prepared and followed. Caution must be exercised to avoid dominance of the meeting by members of the union organizing committee. Management must demonstrate its ability to maintain firm discipline and yet relate effectively to those who support management as well as those who do not. If possible, let the union organizing committee members discredit themselves in the eyes of the other employees.

During the remainder of the campaign week, supervisors will:

- Stress the ways in which management works toward the security of the employees. A job description provides security by letting employees know what is expected. Performance standards and performance evaluation give security by identifying weaknesses in the employee's performance so that improvements can be made and all benefits realized. The personnel policy manual provides the security of a written statement of the rules, regulations, benefits, and privileges. The employee's economics are made secure through protection of his wage during illness, continuation of income after retirement, and avoidance of medical and hospitalization costs in the event of hospitalization. Continuing education and in-service training protect employees from becoming obsolete due to job changes and new equipment. It is important to stress that the facility is interested in employee security in more ways than one.

- Raise doubts in the employees' minds that the union is equally concerned about employee security.

- Raise questions in the employees' minds as to what would be the realistic next step by the union if, in negotiations, we took a firm position against some union promise and demand. Tell the employees they might be obligated to participate in a work slowdown or stoppage, to take picket duty, or to strike, and that they might be restricted from crossing a picket line to return to their jobs and care directly or indirectly for the patients.

Record and Report: It is important to continue maintaining the one-on-one list of "Yes," "Uncertain" and "No" votes so that at any point there is an updated list available by which to ascertain strengths or weaknesses. The supervisor must maintain continuing notes on interviews, conferences, questions, and problems.

Do You Support the Union or Does the Union Support You?

So much has been said and thought about how the union supports the employee. You might think that the union is here to rescue you from the evils of management. Actually YOU ARE THE TARGET of the union campaign. The union wants you. Examine carefully this list to show how you support the union in contrast to how the union supports you.

HOW YOU SUPPORT THE UNION:

- New member loyalty oath.

- Forfeit your voice to the union representative.

- Submerge personal needs for union position.

- Support activities of other unions with money, time, and effort.

- Pay union assessments for its fines, building programs, political action programs, and welfare plans.

- Required attendance at union meetings.

- Support strikes, take picket duty, and participate in union demonstration.

- Contribute to the cost of arbitration.

- Pay the wages and expense accounts for union leaders, officers, and staff.

- Assume responsibilities as stewards or union officers.

- Pay initiation fees and monthly dues.

- Support union-made products and union-produced services.

HOW THE UNION SUPPORTS YOU:

- Promised wage increases limited in negotiation to what we can pay.

- Promised better benefits if you are willing to strike to get them.

- Improve your work relationships by an organized confrontation with management.

- Allow you to ratify your collective bargaining agreement subject to approval of the international union.

- Give you local voice in determining your collective bargaining procedures subject to the jurisdiction of the international president.

- Provide for your contribution to the strike fund to benefit you when the international union approves.

- Recognize your human dignity while at the same time providing that you may be charged, fined, or reprimanded by the union for infraction of its rules.

THIS IS SOMETHING FOR YOU TO THINK ABOUT!

The Patient: The Innocent Victim

Although we know and express without reservation that we are all here to serve the patient, is it not ironic that through both present and anticipated activities that very patient could become the innocent victim. The facility needs unity, not a union. What handicaps or hurts the facility in like manner hampers our efforts to deliver appropriate care and service to its patients. Let us share some of our thoughts and concerns.

The patient may be the innocent victim when management and the employees find themselves on different

teams, more willing to confront one another than to cooper-
ate within the singular objective--care of the patient.

- **The patient may be the innocent victim when** management personnel and employees must give time to union-related activities--the organizing campaign, the NLRB election, the collective bargaining process, the preparation for
and follow-up after arbitrations--all time that could have
been used to improve patient care and employee relations.

- **The patient may be the innocent victim when** the cost of
patient care services must be increased so that the union
can receive, without penalty to the employees, payment for
its initiation fees, dues, assessments, and other funds for
operational purposes--all of which eventually must come
from the patient without any benefit to the patient, us, or
you.

- **The patient may be the innocent victim when** contracts
must be negotiated to meet the needs of the union--cer-
tainly not the needs of the patients, not ours, and seldom
even your needs.

- **The patient may be the innocent victim when** management's rights have been eroded through collective bargaining, which may place the union in a position for review, appeal, or even arbitration on matters that affect the
rights to hire; fire; determine the job and assignments without conflict of job jurisdiction; establish performance standards; conduct performance appraisal, exercising corrective
action or granting reward and recognition where appropriate; modify procedures, methods, or technological improvements in the interest of better patient care without
union intervention; modify wages, benefits, or personnel
policies as conditions permit in the interest of improved
employee relations to indirectly stimulate patient care; and
staff and schedule employees when and where needed to
meet patient care needs.

- **The patient may be the innocent victim when** non-health
care oriented representatives attempt to negotiate conditions that determine how the facility may operate when
both management and the employees know better and when

they care and work cooperatively to improve operational practice in the interest of good patient care.

- **The patient may be the innocent victim when** good and capable workers are unwilling to work at a facility that is unionized, causing good workers to terminate their employment and handicapping recruitment of other workers--which further complicates and handicaps the delivery of service and care to the patients. Keep in mind that three out of four workers in the American labor force are NOT UNION.

- **The patient may be the innocent victim when** there are work interruptions by slowdowns, stoppages, or strikes, or when the union interferes with operations through pickets, picket lines, and control of deliveries of needed supplies.

EXPRESS CARE, INC. NEEDS UNITY--NOT A UNION. DO NOT BE MISLED. IF THE EMPLOYEES AND MANAGEMENT WORK TOGETHER, WE CAN PROTECT THE PATIENT FROM BECOMING THE INNOCENT VICTIM.

Guide for Supervisors: Week 4-- The Week Before or of the Election

Objective: It is the intention of this final week campaign to influence every employee to vote in the NLRB election and to vote ''No.'' It is intended that all union propaganda issues be countered so that employees have a legitimate position to counter every union position. During this final week we need to recap and reinforce all of our major positions. The ultimate target is for 100 percent of the employees to vote and get a decisive rejection of the union, and thereby prevent a recurrence of the union organizing effort a year hence or an effort from an opposing union.

Supervisory Support: The continuing pattern of a close one-to-one relationship of supervisors with employees must be maintained. By this time you and the employees should have a friendly and personal relationship with at least basic mutual respect and understanding. The key assumption at this point is that employees will not vote for the union if they have a good relationship with their immediate supervisors.

Communication Guideline: In this final week of the election campaign, supervisors should be extremely sensitive to those employees who are hard-core unionists in contrast to those who are hard-core for the facility. It is now too late for the union to persuade the loyal employees to vote union, but it is equally too late for the facility to persuade the hard-core union employees to vote for the institution. Therefore, time and effort should be concentrated on the employees who remain on the "uncertain" list. A number of specific points should be pursued:

- The unconcerned or uninvolved employees must be made aware that if they fail to vote and the union does win the election, they would be involved, as far as the union is concerned, in the resulting collective bargaining agreement, conditions, restrictions, and benefits. To remain uninvolved, such employees must vote "No" in sufficient numbers to assure the union defeat.

- The election is absolutely by secret ballot. Advise the employee to clearly place the X within the square under the word "No" and not to sign the ballot or make any other marks on it. (See Exhibit 3.)   The ballot should be folded and placed in the ballot box personally by the employee.

- Based on working schedules, attempt without open discrimination to have all of the uncertain employees scheduled on duty the day of the election to minimize inconvenience that might be related to their votes. For every hard-core union vote not scheduled on duty, be sure there is a hard-core institution vote also not scheduled on duty so as to avoid any unfair labor practice charges of discrimination.

- The 24-hour rule provides that the day before the election no new issue can be brought to the attention of the employees since it would not offer the other party the opportunity of response. It is now too late for new ideas.

- In the final 24-hour period do not initiate any positions with the employees, but be available to respond to any employee questions or concerns. Respond by reference to materials already made available, positions taken, letters sent, or meetings held.

TIME TO DECIDE YOUR FUTURE

You will decide _your_ future tomorrow. The way you mark your _secret_ ballot may be one of the most important decisions you will make in your life. It can affect _you_, your _family_ and your _future._ You know that we have a good place to work. Let's not turn it over to the Union!

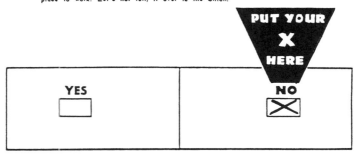

YES

PUT YOUR
X
HERE

NO

YOU HAVE COMPARED THE FACTS —
NOW YOU KNOW THE TRUTH

THE UNION	YOUR EMPLOYER
★ STRIKES	★ A STEADY JOB
★ DUES, FEES, FINES	★ GOOD PAY with NO UNION DUES
★ WILD PROMISES	★ MANY EMPLOYEE BENEFITS
★ UNION BOSSES	★ CHANCE TO GET AHEAD ON MERIT
★ CAN'T TALK FOR YOURSELF	★ FAIR TREATMENT

YOU MAY LOSE A LOT WITH A UNION!

VOTE NO   *VOTE NO*

Exhibit 3

- On the day of the election stay away from the polling booth to avoid unfair labor practice charges. Do not escort any employees to the polling place. The union can do that--but management cannot. Express confidence that the employee has understood the matter and will vote to support us. Smile. Be pleasant.

- Review all log material recorded and reported to determine if there is anything that might be used as a basis for an unfair labor practice charge against the union in the event the union wins the election.

- In the event that we win the election, do not gloat and do not discriminate between those for the institution and those for the union. Simply express appreciation to all employees for a wise decision.

- If the union should win the election, do not criticize, challenge, or condemn the employees. The better response is an expression of hope that this will prove to be the right decision.

Record and Report: Submit your summary and facts regarding any possible unfair labor practice to the Vice-President--Personnel. There is a limit of 5 days after the election when all such charges must be officially filed with NLRB. Do not delay. Thank you and good luck.

We appreciate all the cooperation and support you gave in support of Express Care, Inc. in its efforts to remain a nonunion health care facility.

Management and the Employees Need to be United-- We do not Need a Union

Have you ever considered the real relationship that must exist between you, as an employee, and management? We must work together as ONE TEAM. We must communicate to understand each other and we must trust in order to accept each other. We are the heads and tails of the same coin. Reading from left to right, think about these important relationships.

HOW YOU NEED MANAGEMENT	HOW MANAGEMENT NEEDS YOU
A job and job description.	Performance and quality service.
A justifiable wage and good benefits.	A worker who is worthy of his hire.
Assignments and work schedules	Attendance--on time.
Tools and equipment.	Proper care and use of tools.
Supplies and materials.	Avoid waste.
Patients to assure your job.	To project a positive image.
Orientation, training, and continuing education.	Willingness to assume greater responsibilities.
Organized work with defined procedures, methods, and performance standards.	Achievement of performance standards.
Performance evaluation.	Effective improvement as a health care worker and as a person.
Opportunities to learn.	Application of new ideas to the job performance.
Qualified and appropriate supervision.	Cooperation with management.
Capable fellow employees.	Support of our reputation as a good employer.
Understanding and listening ear.	Employee support in decision making and problem solving.
Administrative team that knows and understands the new economics of the health care industry.	Help us to develop new health care markets to enhance job security.

This list could go on and on showing how many ways you need management and management needs you. There is need for unity--not union. There is need for cooperative team effort--not organized opposition. There is need for our common pursuit of common objectives. We cannot be independent. We dare not be dependent. We are interdependent.

THIS IS SOMETHING FOR YOU TO THINK ABOUT!

What is your Guarantee?

From your experience as an employee of this facility, your personnel policy handbook, your relationships with your supervisor, the past pattern of wage increases and benefit improvements and job security, you know your guarantees from us. A critical issue now is: What is your guarantee from the union?

We suggest that you confront the union organizer and test if you can get a signed guarantee to the following conditions. We believe these are important to your security and to your future.

1. I Guarantee: You will get a pay raise of _____ cents an hour in our very first contract with Express Care, Inc., or my union will be liable.

2. I Guarantee: My union will give you your regular rate of pay beginning the first day you are on strike, or my union will be liable.

3. I Guarantee: There will be absolutely no fines or assessments of any kind against you by my union. If there are, my union should be sued.

4. I Guarantee: There will be no reductions in force or layoffs. If there are, the union will be liable.

5. I Guarantee: My union will pay for your family's support and all of their expenses if you are thrown out of work because of a union strike or shutdown.

6. I Guarantee: Union stewards and union officials will not receive special treatment over you in the event layoffs are

made in your facility by your management, or my union will be liable.

7. I Guarantee: Once you become a member of my union, you will not be required to follow the Constitution and By-laws of my union, or the union will be liable.

8. I Guarantee: If you are called out on strike, you will get your job back at the end of the strike, or my union will be liable.

Signed_____ Date_____

Sworn before me this _____ day of _____
                      (Date)   (Month)

19___ at _____
        (City)   (State)

_____

(Notary)

AFFIX NOTARY SEAL

BIBLIOGRAPHY

HEALTH CARE INDUSTRY--NEW HORIZONS AND ENVIRONMENTS

Bice, M. O. "Corporate Cultures and Business Strategy: A Health Management Company Perspective." *Hospital and Health Services Administration* 29 (July-August 1984): 64-78.

Bills, S. S. "In Crowded Market, Hospital Looks to Wellness for Competitive Edge." *Promoting Health* 5 (January-February 1984): 1-3.

Ellwood, P. M., Jr. "When MDs Meet DRGs." *Hospitals* 57 (December 16, 1983): 62-66.

Griffith, J. R. "The Role of Blue Cross and Blue Shield in the Future U.S. Health Care System." *Inquiry* 20 (Spring 1983): 12-19.

Hearne, T. "Managing Public Opinion in a Hostile Environment." *HMQ Hospital Management Quarterly* (Spring 1984): 7-11.

Johnson, D. E. L. "For-Profits Join Nonprofits on New Deals." *Modern Healthcare* 13 (June 1983): 42.

Kahn, L. "Meeting of the Minds." *Hospitals* 57 (March 1983): 84-86.

Littlefield, J. E. "Home Health Care: The Opportunity for Health Care Marketing." *Journal of Health Care Marketing* 4 (Winter 1984): 51-55.

MacStravic, R. S. "Persuasive Communication Strategies for Hospitals." *Health Care Management Review* 9 (Spring 1984): 69-75.

Nystrom, P. C. "Managing Beliefs in Organizations." *The Journal of Applied Behavioral Science* 20 (1984): 277-287.

Pascale, T. "Fitting New Employees Into the Company Culture." *Fortune* 109 (May 28, 1984): 28-30±.

Ramage, R. C. "United We Stand; Divided the Outcome is Less Clear." *Trustee* 36 (Sept. 1983): 19-20, 22, 23.

Strum, A. C., Jr. "Selling the Medical Staff and Hospital as a Package." *Hospitals* 58 (May 16, 1984): 98-101.

Ting, H. M. "New Directions in Nursing Home and Home Health-care Marketing. *Healthcare Financial Management* 38 (May 1984): 62-72.

White, J. S. "How Your New Competitors Plan to Leave You in the Dust." *Medical Economics* 61 (February 20, 1984): 242-249, 252-253.

HEALTH CARE INDUSTRY LABOR RELATIONS

Bloem, R. S. "Collective Bargaining: What's It All About and What Can It Do For You?" *Journal of Practical Nursing* 25 (March, April 1975): 25-26.

Brody, P. E., and London, J. "How Costly Is a Strike?" *Hospitals* 49 (September 16, 1975): 53.

Despres, L. M. "What the National Labor Relations Act Says." *American Journal of Nursing* 76 (May 1976): 790.

Elkin, R. D. "Negotiating and Administering a Union Contract." *Hospital Progress* 56 (January 1975): 40.

Emanuel, W. J. "Coping with the National Labor Relations Act: A Checklist." *Hospital Forum* 17 (November 1974): 15.

Emanuel, W. J., and Klein, A. "Solicitation Rules Will Need Revision." *Hospitals* 49 (August 16, 1975): 47.

Epstein, R. L. "Dare you Say How You Feel About Unionization?" *Trustee* 28 (January 1975): 17.

_____. "Guide to National Labor Relations Board Rules on Solicitation and Distribution." *Hospitals* 49 (August 16, 1975): 43.

_____. "National Labor Relations Board Bargaining Unit Decisions." *Trustee* 28 (July 1975): 79.

Epstein, R. L., and Stickler, K. B. "Nurse as a Professional and as a Unionist." *Hospitals* 50 (January 16, 1976): 44.

Henig, R. M. "Nurses Face Tomorrow: New Power, New Roles, New Problems." *The New Physician* 25 (May 1976): 28.

Laliberty, Rene, and Joseph J. Bean, Jr. *Understanding Hospital Labor Relations.* Reading, MA: Addison-Wesley, 1977.

Packer, C. L. *Preparing Hospital Management for Labor Contract Negotiations.* Chicago: American Hospital Association, 1975.

Pointer, P. D., and Metzger, N. *The National Labor Relations Act: A Guidebook for Health Care Administrators.* New York: Spectrum Publications, Inc., 1975.

Rayworth, J. F. "Final Offer Selection: A Solution to Labor Impasses?" *Hospital Administration in Canada* 16 (September 1974): 58.

Shershin, M. J., and Boxx, W. R. "Building Positive Union-Management Relations." *Personnel Journal* 54 (January 1975): 326.

Usery, W. J., Jr. "Work of the Federal Mediation and Conciliation Service (Interview)." *Hospitals* 48 (September 16, 1974): 45.

PERSONNEL PRACTICES FOR THE '80s

American Hospital Association. *Employee-Labor Relations in Health Care Institutions*. Chicago: AHA, 1975.

Bean, Joseph J., Jr., and Rene Laliberty. *Decentralizing Hospital Management*. Reading, MA: Addison-Wesley, 1980.

Bennett, Addison, C. *Improving Management Performance in Health Care Institutions*. Chicago: American Hospital Association, 1978.

Christopher, W. I., and Rene Laliberty. *Enhancing Productivity in Health Care Facilities*. Owings Mills, MD: National Health Publishing, 1984.

Conklin, William E., Jr. *A Basic Guide to Health Care Personnel Policies and Procedures*. Chicago: American Society for Hospital Personnel Administration, 1985.

_____. "Employee Relations." *Hospitals* 49 (April 1, 1975): 75.

American Society for Hospital Personnel Administration. *Fair Shakes: The Health Care Compensation Hand-Book*. Chicago: American Society for Hospital Personnel Administration, 1984.

INDEX

conflict, 38-39
growth, 5-6, 11, 12
sicker patient trend, 11, 12
Nursing service, work stoppage, 110

Occupational Safety and Health Act,
    37, 118
Occupational Safety and Health
    Review Commission, 33
Organization
    authoritarian, 7
    democratic, 7
    formal, 7
Orientation, 128, 129, 138
Outpatient center, 218
Outsider, 69-72
    disruptive demonstration, 119
    solicitation and distribution, 73

Paternalism, 16
Patient care
    area, 73
    unionization effects, 257-258
    during work stoppage, 67
Patient census, decrease, 217-218
    during work stoppage, 107, 108,
        114, 115
Payment system
    cost-based, 10-11
    fixed-price, 10
    Prospective. *See* Prospective
    Payment System.
Pension, 34
Performance
    evaluation, 139
    substandard, 95
Performance standard, 84, 126, 128,
    139, 198
    unfair evaluation, 162
    union effects, 56
    unrealistic, 161-162

Personnel
    governing board responsibility, 41
    skills assessment, 112
Personnel department
    answering service, 174
    computer records, 141-143
    governing board, 49
    internal audit
        checklist, 207
        measurement standards, 206
        report, 206
    scope, 137-141
    staff caliber, 206, 207
Personnel director, 50, 134-135
    personnel program, 127
Personnel management, 43, 123, 125-
    137
    department head, 127
    goal, 126, 127
    philosophy, 125
    supervisor, 127
Personnel policy, 84, 94, 208
    distribution, 148
    format, 148-153
    inconsistent enforcement, 158
    initiation, 151
    legal review, 145
    need for, 148
    problems due to, 148
    procedures, 149, 152
    purpose, 149
    responsibility, 149, 151-152
    review, 151-153
Personnel program, 43-50, 125-137
    evaluation, 132-133
    goals, 207
    management controls, 141
    professional audit, 84
Personnel record, 83-84, 133-134,
    138, 211
    standardized, 134
Physician
    authority, 8